T0221248

AN APPROACH TO THE
PSYCHOLOGY OF RELIGION

Founded by C. K. Ogden

The International Library of Psychology

ANTHROPOLOGY AND PSYCHOLOGY
In 6 Volumes

AN APPROACH TO THE PSYCHOLOGY OF RELIGION

J CYRIL FLOWER

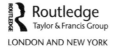

Routledge
Taylor & Francis Group

LONDON AND NEW YORK

First published in 1927
by Routledge, Trench, Trubner & Co., Ltd

Reprinted in 1999, 2000, 2001 (twice)
by Routledge
2 Park Square, Milton Park, Abingdon, Oxon, OX14 4RN

Simultaneously published in the USA and Canada by Routledge

711 Third Avenue, New York, NY 10017

Transferred to Digital Printing 2007

Routledge is an imprint of the Taylor & Francis Group

First issued in paperback 2013

© 1927 J Cyril Flower

British Library Cataloguing in Publication Data
A CIP catalogue record for this book
is available from the British Library

An Approach to the Psychology of Religion

ISBN 978-0-415-20951-9 (hbk)
ISBN 978-0-415-86433-6 (pbk)

CONTENTS

v

INTRODUCTION

THE following chapters contain the substance of a Cambridge Ph.D. Dissertation submitted by me in 1925, entitled *The Bearing of Recent Developments of Psychological Study upon Religion*. In offering the volume for publication I prefer to do so under a more modest title, but the Introduction I wrote for the original work is still the most suitable I can write for introducing this book to its readers. The title of the Dissertation, accepted by the Board of Research Studies as a general indication of the field of research I desired to undertake, embraces so large an area that it was obviously necessary to select within it some specific problem for detailed consideration and treatment. In the course of general observation and special investigation I became impressed with the importance for any psychological account of religion of the recent development of the concept of active ' tendencies ' as determining influences in behaviour. Accordingly, it is with the bearing of this development of psychological study upon religion that I have almost exclusively concerned myself The connection between religious practice and belief on the one hand, and instinct together with other original or innate ' tendencies ' of a more individual character on the other hand is, in a general way, obvious. But the attempts made by various writers to derive religion from any one instinct or group of instincts, seemed to me to fail to account for many of the characteristic features of the religious response.

vii

The idea occurred to me that the widespread phenomena of religion, both in connection with practice and belief, might be connected with original tendencies not directly, as immediate, distorted or sublimated expressions of their operation either singly or in co-operation, but indirectly, as the result of their failure to function in the presence of an ever increasing discrimination of features in the environment which provided no adequate stimulus to them.

This is the leading idea which I have tried to establish and expound in the chapters which follow. It appeared to me on general grounds to be a fact, patent to observation, that there are differences in the extent of discrimination, and that these differences of discriminative capacity constitute one of the most important distinctions between the mentality of the lower forms of life and that of the higher. Roughly speaking, the wider the area of discrimination, the more complex is the mental life as displayed in adaptive and purposive behaviour. Accepting the point of view of mental evolution it is clear that between the mentality of organisms with fixed and narrow discriminative capacity and those which display a wider range of this capacity, there must be transition. While it is impossible to give any account in terms of inner experience of the transition periods in animal life, it is possible to give some account of it in human life, for every one of us actually makes transition from stage to stage, and some of the transitional periods, at least, occur at a time when there is the power of self observation. My first point, then, is that the universe to which the organism is related grows in extent as we ascend the scale of mental life, and that the effect of a more fully discriminated world upon the mental life of the organism related to it must be of vital importance.

On the supposition that mentality in general means capacity to respond effectively to stimulus, and that such capacity in the earlier phases of life is innate, and existent in the form of tendencies for more or less specific reaction, it is clear that something very important and influential happens if and when an organism so endowed for practical and active purposes, finds itself faced with a situation in which it is capable of discriminating something more than what is adequate stimulus to the innate tendencies.

It is not possible to adduce evidence to shew directly what such an experience involves at the period of transition from immediately pre-human to human mentality, but it seems justifiable to maintain that it will have far-reaching results, and that they will be results which will continue to function and will differentiate man from his pre-human ancestors. What these results are I have endeavoured to trace in the text. In an Appendix (page 211) I have suggested in a very tentative manner the possible dawn of religious behaviour ; but I do not place much value on this attempt.

A more direct method of testing the theory that religion from the psychological point of view is one of the major results of the enormous extension of the universe discriminated by man—a discrimination altogether in excess of his innate tendencies for direct response—seemed to me to be afforded by the fact that this discrimination is not a solitary event, but a continuous process. Accordingly any careful investigation of the process of religious development, and of new religious outburst, should reveal the operation of what I have called the ' frustration ' experience. I have followed this clue in the argument of my book, the general plan of which may now be outlined.

In the first and second chapters I have tried to state and particularize as clearly as possible the theory I desire to advance as a principle of psychological interpretation. In the third and fourth chapters I have considered the valuable material presented by Dr. Paul Radin concerning the religion of the Winnebago Indians, and the introduction among them of the Peyote Cult, and I have sought to shew that this illustrates the operation of precisely the ' frustration experience ' which I have maintained as psychologically fundamental. It has been a great encouragement to me to have Dr. Radin's expression of approval of and agreement with my interpretation and use of this material. The fifth chapter consists of an analysis of the experience of George Fox, as recorded in his *Journal;* and in this instance, again, I believe that the theory I have advanced makes possible a fuller understanding of the psychological nature of the religion of the founder of Quakerism. Chapter VI is a brief account of some of the salient features of the conversion experience in general, as a particular expression of the frustration experience. The concluding chapter on Religion and Psychopathology is chiefly concerned with a recent attempt on the part of Dean Everett Martin to give an account of religion in terms of psychopathology. In criticizing this attempt I have endeavoured to shew that the method of approach I have advocated places the valuable contributions of psychopathology in a fuller and truer context.

I have added three Appendices. The first, as already noted, is an attempt to indicate how prehistoric art in certain cases, if it is religious material, may be interpreted in the light of the frustration experience. The second is a critical note on Rudolf Otto's *The Idea of the Holy,* which seemed to me to require fuller notice than it had received in the text of the book. The third deals very briefly with some of the responses to a questionnaire I issued early in the course of my research. It was of rather a general character, and I have limited my references to those questions which seemed to me to bear directly on the issues involved in this inquiry.

With regard to my use of authorities : I have exercised great care in the endeavour to make full references in footnotes and otherwise to all authors and their works from whom I have quoted, and to whom I am indebted for a particular fact or opinion. But in fact the extent of my indebtedness to writers on the subjects which come within the purview of this book is far wider than it has been possible specifically to record. I know that the general direction of my psychological investigations and thought have been largely influenced by the following, who have been, at various periods, my teachers and whose lectures and classes I attended : Dr. W. R. Boyce Gibson, Prof. L. T. Hobhouse, Dr. E. Westermarck ; the late Dr. W. H. R. Rivers, under whose supervision I commenced my research at Cambridge, and for whose sympathy and encouragement in the few months I came under his influence I owe a very great deal ; Mr. F. C. Bartlett, Dr. G. Dawes Dicks, and Mr. J. T. MacCurdy, who supervised my research after the death of Dr. Rivers.

THE PSYCHOLOGY OF RELIGION

I

WHAT IS RELIGION?

IT has been said that 'definitions of psychology must express direction rather than delimitation', and it may be safely asserted that the same principle holds in the case of religion—if indeed any definition at all is to be attempted —for as numerous writers[1] have pointed out, the name has

[1] Thus William James, in *The Varieties of Religious Experience*, 30th Impression, 1919, on p. 26, says : '. . . the word " religion " cannot stand for any single principle or essence, but is rather a collective name. . . . Let us not fall immediately into a one-sided view of our subject, but let us rather admit freely at the outset that we may very likely find no one essence, but many characters which may alternately be equally important in religion.'

Sir James G. Frazer, in *The Golden Bough*, London, 1913, Vol. I, p. 222, says : 'There is probably no subject in the world about which opinions differ so much as the nature of religion, and to frame a definition of it which would satisfy every one must obviously be impossible. All that a writer can do is, first, to say clearly what he means by religion, and afterwards to employ the word consistently in that sense throughout his work.'

J. B. Pratt, in *The Religious Consciousness*, New York, 1921, p. 1, says : 'The truth is, I suppose, that " religion " is one of those general and popular terms which have been used for centuries to cover so vague and indefinite a collection of phenomena that no definition can be framed which will include all its uses and coincide with every one's meaning for it. Hence all definitions of religion are more or less arbitrary and should be taken rather as postulates than as axioms.'

R. H. Thouless, in *An Introduction to the Psychology of Religion*, 1923, p. 4, after formulating a definition, goes on to say : 'This definition will be found to be sufficient for the purpose for which we require it—to indicate the sense in which the word *religion* will be used in the course of this book. Possibly for a different purpose, a different definition would have been found more convenient.'

Such quotations could, of course, be indefinitely multiplied. But while this note of caution is a salutary reminder of the difficulties and pitfalls in the search for definitions in religion, I think there is urgent need for the attempt to formulate a genetic definition, which will bring out the threads of continuity and identity connecting all the types of behaviour and experience, ancient and modern, savage, ' primitive ', and civilized, which we call ' religious '.

been given to so great a variety of expressions of behaviour and experience that it is exceedingly difficult to formulate an accurate and clear-cut definition which covers them all. At the outset it is of importance to emphasize certain broad facts concerning religion as the subject matter of psychological inquiry. Religion as we commonly use the word, stands for at least two distinguishable things : (i) Behaviour as actually observable, and (ii) Experience, which may or may not issue in behaviour which is observable. Religion as predominantly observable behaviour finds expression in the course of development in such things as ceremony, ritual and conventional observances. Religion as experience has to do with the individual as such, and may be confined to an inner life of which no outsider has any direct knowledge. There it may take two characteristic forms, (a) cognitive—the acceptance or formulation of beliefs ; and (b) affective—the most striking type of which is what is known as mystical experience. Some of the mystics have endeavoured to give expression to their inner experience in verbal form—and of course the general behaviour of many of them has been an obvious expression of the forces of an inward experience—but it is exceedingly difficult for any one who has not in some measure participated in mystical experience to appreciate the meaning of mystical writings as the expression of a definitely affective conscious experience. In some instances a certain amount of light has been shed upon the psychological mechanisms of the mystic's experience by analytic psychology and psychopathology.[1]

[1] Janet, *Major Symptoms of Hysteria*, 1907, Lect. I ; C. G. Jung, *Collected Papers on Analytical Psychology*, 1917, ch. i ; *Psychology of the Unconscious*, 1919; *Psychological Types*, 1923. R. H. Thouless, *op. cit.*, chs. xv and xvi. Th. Flournoy, *Une Mystique Moderne* (Archives de Psychologie, Tome xv), 1915. Wm. James, *Varieties of Religious Experience*, Lect. I.

The distinction between the two references of the word may be brought out more clearly and emphasized by an illustration. If we see a man enter a church, pass in front of the altar, and bow or cross himself, we might say that he has performed a religious act. But we could not proceed to assert that he was a religious person, for his behaviour might have been due to motives which had no religious significance ; he might, for instance, have entered the church as an interested student of architecture, and seeing other people genuflecting before the altar, wished to fall in with prevailing customs. But if we found that the man not only performed the act, but, when asked, gave an account of his act in terms of certain inner experiences and beliefs, we should then say that he was a religious man.

But a further piece of verbal analysis of a preliminary character has to be carried out. The adjective ' religious ' has an even wider reference than the substantive ' religion'. An act may be called religious, though performed by a person who is not religious—that is to say, apart from all questions of personal attitude. A person may be called religious by reason of inner experience, whether or not they are expressed in observable behaviour : these two usages corresponding with the distinction made between religion as behaviour and as experience. But in addition certain things, places, times—in fact anything which can be psychological material—may under certain circumstances come to be spoken of as ' religious '. All objects which are directly connected with religious behaviour or religious experience are, so far forth, called religious. Thus we speak of religious buildings, religious utensils, religious vestments, religious seasons, religious feasts, fasts, and so forth. This attachment of a religious quality to objects is of extreme psychological interest and importance, and is intimately connected with the origin of religious behaviour. Religious behaviour is response of a more or less particular kind to objects which are treated as religious. Which comes first, the religious behaviour, or the recognition of an independent ' religiousness ' in the object or situation responded to ? The intrinsic religiousness of certain objects or situations is a problem for religious philosophy, and no doubt a quite fundamental problem. The rock upon which most religious philosophy splits when it tries to demonstrate the ' intrinsic ' religiousness of certain things is, of course, the fact that the adjective religious is applied to such various and diverse objects. The problem of the psychology of religion is a different one, and may thus be stated : Can we trace the psychological conditions which give to certain situations or objects a religious value in the estimation of the persons concerned, quite apart from the question whether there is a specific religious nature in these, or any other objects at all ?

The primary thing with which we are concerned is religious behaviour—that is, response of a certain peculiar character to a situation, or objects in a situation, of a certain kind. We may—indeed as I think we must— consider this in the first instance without having in mind any conception of self-conscious insight or purpose. The guiding concept, familiar in modern psychology, is that behaviour precedes all self-awareness in behaving. Evolutionary psychology seeks to trace the growth of behaviour from the *adaptive* stage to the self-conscious and purposive ; and it is extremely difficult to draw any hard and fast line, and say that before this all is mere *adaptivity*, and after this we are in the realm of *purposiveness* as a fact of self-consciousness. It is quite possible, even probable, in the light of general principles, that man began to behave religiously (according to my terminology) before he was capable of having any definite awareness and appreciation of the inner side of the behaviour. This point is of sufficient importance to justify further elucidation, before I proceed to the main stream of the discussion.

When we speak of religious behaviour we may, as has been pointed out, mean behaviour which is regarded by the observer as religious because it conforms to the established conventions of people who so act in order to give expression to some sort of religious experience. On the other hand we may mean behaviour which is peculiar, but which we have reason to know is, for the person concerned, conditioned by his particular religious experience. This is constantly illustrated in common speech. A man who makes no profession of any kind, takes no part in any sort of religious ceremony or worship, and asserts that he does not share any of the beliefs ordinarily associated with religion, is nevertheless often described by those who know him best as a *deeply* or *essentially religious man*. What is meant in attributing religion in such a case is that the persons making the judgment consider that the general behaviour, or way of life, of that man is of the kind which would normally be the outcome of his being religious in the more conventional sense, and on the principle ' by their fruits ye shall know them ', do not hesitate to postulate religion as an unrecognized, or unconscious motive. Religion, that is to say, is often attributed on the basis of being and doing, and not solely on the basis of believing and behaving through conventional forms and ceremonies. Now when we are dealing with savage races, and still more when we

are trying to reconstruct the psychology of ' primitive '
man,[1] we are not justified in assuming the existence of
conscious motives similar to those which we introspect in
ourselves. Accordingly, if we characterize certain kinds
of response as being religious, what we mean is that they
are responses which we can see to have essential characteristics in common with that mass of responses which at a
more developed stage are accompanied by some conscious
religious reference. We have no right to assume that
' primitive ' man was sufficiently aware of himself to interpret his own responses, or to make the clear-cut ideational
discriminations which seem natural to us ; and when we
do so we probably effect a rationalization which may be
quite misleading. Let us consider an instance. It is
frequently assumed[2] that Mousterian man believed in ' life
after death ' because of the evidence of burial of the dead.
Thus Prof. J. Y. Simpson[3] says :

> ' The most objective evidence of the religious beliefs of Mous-
> terian man is connected with the burial of his dead. The facts
> seem to express a belief in some sort of a future existence that was
> a continuation of the present. Food was placed beside the
> traveller—for only slowly did the spirit extricate itself from its
> tenement of clay—and his flint implements and ornaments, or
> it may be the most prized ones of those who were his friends,
> were buried with him ; he would have need of them. The interest
> becomes evidence of real affection when we consider how, as at
> La Ferrassie, flat stones had been laid over the head and shoulders
> as if to protect them, and in the case of the youth buried at Le
> Moustier, the head had been laid on a pillow of flint chippings.'

---

[1] Which is not necessarily the same thing. As R. R. Marett says, in
Anthropology (Home University Library), p. 39 : ' . . . . the Australians,
or Tasmanians, or Bushmen, or Eskimo, of whom so much is beginning to be
heard amongst pre-historians, are our contemporaries—that is to say,
have just as long an ancestry as ourselves ; and in the course of the last
100,000 years or so our stock has seen so many changes, that their stocks
may possibly have seen a few also '.

[2] See R. R. Marett, *op. cit.*, pp. 79-80, 206. Also *Psychology and Folk-
lore*, 1920, pp. 238-9.

[3] *Man and the Attainment of Immortality*, p. 116.

Now, we cannot interrogate Mousterian man ; nor has any Mousterian philosopher left us a discourse on his ' beliefs ' : all we have before us is evidence, in the shape of products and survivals of behaviour. What we infer with assurance is that in certain cases the response of Mousterian man to some situation involving the disposal of the body of a fellow, was the burial of the body with food, implements, etc. Now if *we* did that, we can only imagine ourselves burying persons who were, in the first place, actually dead, and then only if we believed that our dead friend's body, or soul, would need food and tools, and could make use of them in some kind of life after death. Must we assume that Mousterian man acted on the same conscious discriminations and beliefs ?[1] I do not think the evidence is nearly cogent enough to make this inference imperative, or even the most probable. It may be true, but there is another hypothesis which will cover the known facts, and which is in harmony with (and derives support from) contemporary observations. That is to say, these burial practices may have been due to a failure to appreciate the fact of death in the clear-cut fashion in which we recognize it. Before we dismiss this, with Dr. Marett, as a far-fetched

---

[1] Dr. R. R. Marett dismisses the alternative explanation as ' jest '. He says (*Psychology and Folk-Lore*, pp. 238-9) : ' Before we leave the Mousterians, another side of their culture deserves brief mention. Not only did they provide their dead with rude graves, but they likewise furnished them with implements and food for use in a future life. Herein surely we may perceive the dawn of what I do not hesitate to term religion. A distinguished scholar and poet did indeed once ask me whether the Mousterians, when they performed these rites, did not merely show themselves unable to grasp the fact that the dead are dead. But I presume that my friend was jesting. A sympathy stronger than death, over-riding its grisly terror, and converting it into the vehicle of a larger hope—that is the work of soul. . . . ' It is to be noted that in this passage Marett does not state the facts, and then see what can be said about them ; he states the facts in terms of a foregone conclusion about their meaning, and then deduces what he does not hesitate to call religion and the soul. He is then unable to take an alternative interpretation of the facts seriously.

notion, let us attend to important evidence, and its interpretation, supplied by the research of Dr. W. H. R. Rivers.[1]
He says :

'Death is so striking and unique an event that if one had to choose something which must have been regarded in essentially the same light by mankind at all times and in all places, I think one would be inclined to choose it in preference to any other ; and yet I hope to show that the conception of death among such people as the Melanesians is different, one may say radically different, from our own.

'. . . on looking up any Melanesian vocabulary it will be found that some form of the word *mate* is given as the equivalent of dead, and that dead is given as the meaning of *mate*, but as a matter of fact such statements afford most inadequate expression of the real conditions. It is true that the word *mate* is used for a dead man, but it is also used for a person who is seriously ill and likely to die, and also often for a person who is healthy, but so old that, one may suppose from the native point of view, if he is not dead, he ought to be. . . .

'. . . Further, here—as, in my experience, universally in low states of culture—these are not mere verbal categories, but are of real practical importance. Every one has heard of the practice of burying the living, customs well known to have existed in Melanesia ; and I have little doubt in the old days whenever a suitable opportunity arose, those who were called *mate* would have been actually submitted to the funeral rites, which would have made them dead in our sense as well as *mate*. Even now the Melanesians do not wait till a sick man is dead in our sense, but if he is considered sufficiently *mate*, movements or even groans will furnish no grounds for stopping the funeral rites, including among these rites the process of burial ; and a person who, through external interference, is rescued from this predicament, may have a very unpleasant time, for it would seem that nothing would make such a man other than *mate* for the rest of what we call his life.

'We think of burial as a means of disposing of the dead body ; but to primitive man it is possible, I believe even probable, that the matter is not at all regarded in this utilitarian way, but that burial or other means of disposing of the body is to him merely one of the rites suitable to the condition of what I have called *mate*-ness. One of the fundamental fallacies of the anthropologist —I would call it the anthropologists' fallacy, if I were not afraid that it is merely one among many—is to suppose that because a rite or other institution fulfils a certain utilitarian purpose, it

[1] Art. in Hibbert Journal, *The Primitive Conception of Death*, vol. x, No. 2, pp. 397-8.

therefore came into being in order to fulfil that purpose ; and, though it may perhaps seem strained and far-fetched, I am quite prepared to consider whether even such a practice as burial, which seems to have so obvious and utilitarian a purpose, may not really have come into being from some quite different motive.'

In the light of this it is by no means a merely fanciful assertion that Mousterian man may not have been in the habit of burying his dead at all—but may have been in the habit of burying his *mate* (or the Mousterian equivalent), without clearly discriminating between conditions of sickness, trance, death, and old age. And if so, what more natural than that food should be placed near, implements handy, and some measure of comfort in the shape of a flint pillow should be accorded ? Not because of anything so clear-cut as a belief in an ' after life ', but because there is no reason why a *mate* person should not have many needs in common with persons not *mate*. As a matter of behaviour we may regard the fact of burial by Mousterian man as religious ; but the important point is that in describing such phenomena as religious we do not mean that we attribute any particular ideas, beliefs or even clear-cut feelings to the persons so behaving ; we mean by calling the behaviour religious that we detect a close and unmistakable resemblance between the acts performed and the acts of more developed men which are ascertainably connected with religious experience as we can appreciate it. In this sense we may see that it is not impossible that religion as a behaviouristic phenomenon may precede any definite awareness, and it may be that man has come to believe religiously and to feel religiously because in an earlier phase he behaved religiously. In the particular case of early burial, for instance, the fact that man found himself burying his *mate* may have led to the formulation of the belief in life after death, when once the *mate* condition had been more clearly analysed and understood. If the child in any sense recapitulates the story of man's psychological development, we may note as an interesting fact that it is by the habituation of the child in behaviour such as saying prayers at a time when they have no meaning for him, adopting particular postures, attending church or Sunday School, and a variety of other similar habitual acts, that his religious education usually begins. That is to say, in the ordinary case of a child's religious discipline, behaviour precedes and leads up to belief, which in turn influences behaviour, and also behaviour largely helps to condition and define feeling.

Does it not become inevitable, then, to raise the question : To what sort of objects, or to what kind of situation, would man be likely to make a religious response ? The question in that form is only inevitable if we are seeking to indicate the nature of religion by defining a religious response, or religious behaviour, in terms of objects or situations which are held to be intrinsically religious. And in that case it would obviously be necessary to inquire into the question of the characteristics of the objects or situations which constitute them religious. That has been, very largely, the customary method of approach to the problem both by anthropologists and psychologists—influenced probably by the prevalent view of theology that religion is essentially intercourse with supernatural powers. With this idea in mind, some special character or nature of objects in the environment has been singled out which, it is supposed, produced the particular kind of response which is known as religious. An instance of this is afforded by Martineau,[1]

[1] *The Seat of Authority in Religion*, 2nd ed., 1890. pp. 1-3.

who depicts primitive man as projecting life and spirit upon external nature, and discerning

> ' behind the looks and movements of nature, a Mind, that is the seat of power and the spring of every change.'

In the same way many of the prevalent definitions of religion which follow Tylor's ' minimum definition ' [1] seem to assume the discrimination of a special character in the environment which is ' spiritual ' or ' supernatural '. But an empirical study of the facts must lead to a modification of such statements. The whole question of an intrinsic religiousness or a metaphysical supernaturalness is beyond the scope of a psychological inquiry, as I have already insisted. Theological interpretations of experience are neither admitted nor disputed by the psychologist of religion who attends to his own buiness, which is to give a coherent account so far as that may be possible of the behaviour (which in the widest sense includes inner experience) known as religion in terms of the known mechanisms of the mind, and in terms of necessary generalizations concerning its functions as manifest throughout the field of mental life. Now the most obvious fact for the psychologist in this connection is that there is almost no object or situation in the world which may not under certain circumstances have religious significance—that is, primarily, condition religious behaviour. Thus it is evident that it is not so much the situation that has a special character of its own, as it is the responder to the situation who has a special attitude to it ; and psychologically it is this attitude which constitutes religiousness. Thus a man-like ape may

----

[1] *Primitive Culture*, 4th ed., 1903, vol. i, p. 424 : ' It seems best . . . simply to claim, as a minimum definition of religion, the belief in spiritual beings '.

conceivably be surprised in an exposed place by a thunderstorm, and his response may be, under the ' steer ' of an
activated tendency, to seek shelter, and possibly to display
some of the outward marks of fear. So far as his native
preparations for response (which may be roughly lumped for
present purposes as instincts) are called into play and
function effectively, he adapts himself, to the limits of his
determinate capacity, to the situation—and that is the
end of the matter. We may conceive precisely the same
thing happening to the ape-like man. So long as his
instinctive equipment and his environment balance one
another, and there is no dis-proportion between them which
can make itself a further stimulus, he behaves in the kind
of way that can be classified as instinctive ; which from
the present point of view means that he behaves without
giving any indications which can be regarded as having
religious implications. Moreover, it should be noted,
according to a very general theory among psychologists,
who here differ from McDougall,[1] to the extent that this
balance between environmental stimulation and instinctive
response is maintained, there is no experience of emotion.[2]

[1] McDougall maintains that emotion, as felt experience, is the invariable
attendant upon instinctive behaviour. ' We seem justified in believing
that each kind of instinctive behaviour is always attended by some . . .
emotional excitement, however faint, which in each case is specific or
peculiar to that kind of behaviour.' (*Introd. to Social Psychology*, 2nd ed.,
1909, p. 28.) He includes this in his well-known definition of instinct,
which is (among other things) a disposition ' to experience an emotional
excitement of a particular quality upon perceiving ' the object which
touches off the instinct. (p. 29.) This position is also maintained in the
Outline (chap. xi).

[2] Cf. James Drever, *Instinct in Man*, p. 143 : ' So far as the prosecution
of the instinct-interest takes its normal course, and " worthwhileness "
passes normally into " satisfyingness.", through the definite behaviour
provided for by the neural pre-arrangement we call Instinct, when we are
speaking biologically, so far, there is no emotion. But if in any way this
normal prosecution of the instinct-interest is checked, " tension " will
arise, a tension in feeling which is emotion. The difference between this
" tension " and the simple instinct-interest or " worthwhileness " is a

But we know that in the Greek tradition Zeus was inti‑
mately connected with storms and thunder,[1] and in the
Hebrew tradition Yahweh has all the appearance of having
originally been a storm and thunder god of Mount Sinai.[2]
That is to say, at some stage of human development there
was a response to the thunder and storm which was other
than the mere unhampered discharge of energy through
inherited instinct ' patterns ' or ' structure ', and one which
involved a strong emotional experience. Can we in any
measure by analysis get to closer grips with this sort of
response, and detect the element or elements in it which may

difference in the affective consciousness in some respects analogous to the
difference between conception and perception in the cognitive. That is to
say, feeling " tension " represents a further, though secondary, develop‑
ment of affection. None the less it is for experience purely affective.'
    [1] William Smith, *A Smaller Classical Dictionary*, 1862, p. 462, under
' Zeus ', says : ' He is armed with thunder and lightning, and the shaking
of his ægis produces storm and tempest : a number of epithets of Zeus, in
the Homeric poems, describe him as the thunderer, the gatherer of clouds,
and the like.'
    Two instances in the Ninth Book of the Odyssey may be mentioned :
In Line 67 Zeus is described as νεφεληγερέτα Ζευς, ' Zeus the cloud
compeller (or cloud-gatherer). And in Line 552, in connection with the
making of a sacrifice, he is referred to as Ζηνὶ κελαινεφέι, ' to Zeus black
with clouds ' (or cloud-wrapt).
    [2] H. P. Smith, *Old Testament History*, 1903, in summing up the historical
results of the inquiry into the Mosaic period says, p. 72 : ' The God who
sanctioned the alliance and who became a party to it was Yahweh, the
Storm-God of Sinai.' W. H. Bennett, *Old Testament History*, 1909, p. 26,
says : ' There is much to suggest that He (Yahweh) was often thought of
as the god of the thunderstorm and the hurricane.'
    W. Robertson Smith, *The Religion of the Semites*, 1907, p. 118, says :
' . . . long after the establishment of the Hebrews in Canaan, poets and
prophets describe Jehovah, when He comes to help His people, as marching
from Sinai in thundercloud and storm.' Sir J. G. Fraser, *The Golden
Bough*, vol. v, p. 22, footnote 3, says : ' The Hebrews heard in the clap
of thunder the voice of Jehovah, just as the Greeks heard in it the voice of
Zeus and the Romans the voice of Jupiter.' A. B. Davidson, in Article on
God in Hastings' *Dictionary of the Bible*, says, concerning the word Jehovah
or Yahweh, ' The word being pre-historic, its derivation must remain un‑
certain. It has been connected with Arab *hawa*, " to blow " or " breathe "
J" being the god who is heard in the tempest—the storm-god ; or with,
the verb *hawa*, " to fall " (Job 37, 6), in the causative meaning " the
prostrator "—again the lightning-god. . . .' It is interesting to compare
the account in Exodus, ch. 19, specially verses 16-25, with the story in
1 Kings, ch. 19, verses 11 and 12.

have given to the common phenomenon of the thunderstorm a religious character ? I think, without being unduly speculative, we can, and that thereby we may discover the essential psychological mark of religion—that psychological character of the response which is present in the most primitive manifestation of superstition, whether magic, fetishism, or animism, and in the most exalted forms of religious experience.

At no point probably does modern psychology bear with greater directness and significance upon the subject of religion than in its formulations of the mechanisms of response which lie behind and help to condition human behaviour. In last resort the explanation of behaviour is now commonly sought for in terms of instinct and its compounds and conflicts, together with ' individual difference tendencies ', which are commonly recognized by at least one school of psychologists as ultimate forms determining function.[1] Now useful, and indeed unavoidable, as this general working hypothesis is, there are certain grave dangers which we encounter if we begin to multiply instincts and difference tendencies in order to account for the varieties of behaviour. G. C. Field has gone so far as to urge that while the concept of Instinct is useful, its employment in the plural will almost inevitably lead to the fallacy underlying the old ' faculty psychology '.[2] While this seems to me to be an exaggeration of the dangers of the misuse of a valuable working hypothesis, it must be admitted that the process of endowing man with ' instincts ' and ' tendencies ' sufficient to explain all his responses may

---

[1] F. C. Bartlett, *Psychology and Primitive Culture* (1923), p. 3.   Woodworth, *Psychology*, pp. 89-102, 180-4.
[2] Article, *Faculty Psychology and Instinct Psychology*, Mind, N.S. No. 11 9, specially pp. 258-60.

be—and in some quarters actually is—carried to excess, and can only lead into a *cul-de-sac*. This is especially the case in the psychology of religion, when appeal is made to a specific instinct for God or the spiritual.[1] What we need therefore is a cautious and critical use of this method of explanation, always bearing in mind that ' instincts ' and ' tendencies ' are terms of reference to certain facts and are not self-acting entities. Let us be quite clear on this issue. The term ' tendency ' is a mode of reference to the fact that not mere single responses, but co-ordinated and serial responses all more or less related to one another as links in a chain towards some final adjustment, are carried out under certain conditions. Woodworth describes the ten-

---

[1] Reference may be made by way of illustration to two writers on religious psychology, W. R. Inge, and E. D. Starbuck. Inge, in his *Faith and its Psychology*, persistently assumes such an ' instinct ' thus : ' . . . the deep-seated religious instinct ' (p. 42), ' we have maintained that the primary ground of faith is a normal and ineradicable feeling, instinct, or attraction, present in all minds which are not disqualified from having it by peculiarities which we should all agree, probably, in calling defects, a feeling or instinct that behind the world of phenomena there is a world of eternal values, attracting us towards itself.' (p. 53) ' My thesis that the primary ground of Faith is an instinct or faculty which impels us to seek and find God.' (p. 125) ' According to the view which I uphold . . . there is an original, natural bond between God and the human soul. This innate " tendency to God ", as Robert Browning calls it, may be explained or expressed in very various language. To the psychologist, who rightly disclaims the intention of establishing ultimate truth by means of mental science, it is simply a fact of consciousness to be taken note of and analysed as it stands.'

Starbuck is almost equally emphatic in *The Psychology of Religion*, 4th ed., 1914. He says : ' We may turn . . . to the study of the religious instinct in individuals, and discover there its roots, and the law of sequence of its elements from childhood to maturity. This is the work of the psychology of religion.' (p. 4) ' Religion is a life, a deep-rooted instinct. It exists and continues to express itself whether we study it or not. Just as hunger and the desire for exercise still assert themselves whether or not one knows the conditions underlying them, so will one's spiritual nature function and seek objects for its expression even if we are wholly ignorant intellectually of its nature.' (p. 7) ' It is of extreme importance in considering anything so complex and delicate as the religious instinct . . . to stop and observe some of the danger points . . .' (p. 165).

This seems to me to be either an inexcusably loose use of the term instinct—so loose that it sponges clean out any definite meaning—or else an assertion that the religious response admits of no analysis.

dencies as ' *internal* states that *last* for a time and direct action '.[1] Instincts are particular instances of tendency, and denote those tendencies to respond which are innate, and therefore ready to function independently of experience. Thus we have to conceive of instincts as psycho-physical endowments which are potential directors of activity even when they are not actually functioning. This is what McDougall means in regarding instinct as part of mental structure,[2] MacCurdy in treating them as ' reaction patterns ',[3] and Bartlett in including them under ' functional form '.[4] Generally speaking this hypothesis works well over a large part of the field with which pscyhology is concerned, but when applied to man as we know him, there often has to be an immense amount of ingenuity, if not distortion, employed in order to maintain it. For obviously in man instinct-forms have proved to be an inadequate means of adjustment, and new channels of discharge have been invented. What has done it ? Are we to invent a new ' instinct ' *ad hoc* which is to be endowed with just this function ? Is it an instinct, or an original tendency, which achieves sublimation ? Is the control, fusion, inhibition, and manipulation of instincts and tendencies itself an instinctive process ? If these questions are answered in the affirmative, is it not clear that the new instinct or tendency called in to round off the whole scheme is at least so much distinct from the rest that it deserves and requires special treatment and investigation, and is only named instinct to meet the requirements of a special theory ?

---

[1] *Psychology, A Study of Mental Life,* p. 71.
[2] *An Outline of Psychology,* London, 1923, p. 103.
[3] *Problems in Dynamic Psychology,* p. 263, and International Congress of Psychology, 1923, *Proceedings and Papers,* p. 233.
[4] F. C. Bartlett proposes the term Functional Form rather than Structure (unpublished lecture).

We are, indeed, here up against a fundamental problem in evolutionary psychology. Life—and with it what we speak of as mind—is in process of becoming. Its very nature as we know it is movement and change. But science, inevitably, takes it in slices, or sections, and applies certain more or less static terms of explanation. Thus Prof. L. T. Hobhouse[1] says :

> ' Instinct is a product of evolution. It presides at a certain phase, and has, all in due order, its beginning, its rise, its culmination, and its decline.'

This is perhaps as near as we can get when we set out to describe the complex motions of psychic life : but it is none the less the language of abstraction. Thus we cannot help speaking of ' phases ' or stages as if they were really separable segments of psychical development—one stage at which tropism ' presides '; another characterized by reflex action ; yet another dominated by instinct. Yet between these so-called phases or stages there are all the variations and differences that life itself continuously achieves by being in process of becoming. It may be said that tropism in the course of development proves to be an inadequate mode of response, and we detect the products of its break-down in the appearance of reflex action ; and in the same way reflex, in proving inadequate, leads on to instinct. But the important point for present purposes is that instinct also fails, and so far as we can judge, the type of response that life is pressing towards in this break through the ' reaction-patterns ' of instinct as specific adaptation is what we call volition. In point of fact, however, the higher animals, including man, are still only in a transitional phase, and we actually find that the

[1] *Mind in Evolution*, 2nd ed., 1915, p. 67.

instinct patterns continue to direct a large part of behaviour, while volition as yet directs but little.

Bearing these warnings in mind we proceed to the assumption that tracing mental evolution back we should theoretically reach a phase characterized by the dominance of instincts which related the organism in a practical way to the major needs of life.[1] Now so long as the ancestors of man were adapted to their environment adequately and wholly by the mechanisms of the instincts their behaviour would be regular and calculable, and could be classified without reference to religion—as we find it possible to do, e.g., in the case of bees, wasps and ants. But what is characteristic of mammalian evolution is the fact of ' plasticity ' of response—that is, a growing capacity to modify the immediate tendency to respond to a situation by reference to the discrimination in it of a more complex meaning. The relative fixity, and the plasticity of responses can best be shewn in examples. Prof. L. T. Hobhouse,[2] quoting from Lubbock's *Senses of Animals*, records that

---

[1] It is unnecessary here to attempt to specify these, or the instincts which are the inherited tendencies, or dispositions, adapting the organism to them. Probably the most important attempt so far made at classifying and naming the instincts is that of McDougall in *An Introduction to Social Psychology*, 1909, chs. iii and iv. Other references to books in which this problem is dealt with are : W. H. R. Rivers, *Instinct and the Unconscious*, chs. vi and vii ; J. T. MacCurdy, *Problems of Dynamic Psychology*, chs. xviii-xxii ; R. S. Woodworth, *Psychology*, chs. vi and viii. W. Trotter, *Instincts of the Herd in Peace and in War ;* James Drever, *Instinct in Man ;* VIIth Internat. Congress of Psychology, *Proceedings and Papers*, 1924, *The Classification of Instincts*, by J. Drever and E. Jones, pp. 218-231.

[2] *Mind in Evolution*, 2nd ed., 1915, p. 76. The whole of this chapter (vi) on Instinct is relevant here. Prof. Hobhouse distinguishes between plasticity of instinct, and intelligence, though he conisders that ' Intelligence . . . arises within the sphere of instinct '. (p. 101.) It should be noted that McDougall, in the *Outline*, p. 89, refers to the repetition of this experiment by Mr. and Mrs. Peckham (recorded in their *Wasps, Social and Solitary*). He attributes great importance to the fact that these observers were patient enough to continue watching and experimenting until ' the wasp at last omitted the " ritualistic " act, dragged her prey to the opening and, without laying it down, drew it into the nest '. The fact is both interesting and important, but it does not affect the point that the behaviour in question still illustrates the *relative fixity* of instinct.

'. . . A solitary wasp, *Sphex flavipennis*, which provisions its nest with small grasshoppers, when it returns to the cell, leaves the victim outside, and goes down for a moment to see that all is right. During her absence M. Fabre moved the grasshopper a little. Out came the Sphex, soon found her victim, dragged it to the mouth of the cell, and left it as before. Again and again M. Fabre moved the grasshopper, but every time the Sphex did exactly the same thing, until M. Fabre was tired out.'

This doing again and again the same thing in face of a situation which requires a slight alteration of response suggests a fixity of instinct which is in striking contrast with the plasticity observable by any person who has watched the behaviour of an ordinarily intelligent dog. Such an instance as the following is typical :

' When a certain clever dog, carrying a basket of eggs, with the handle in his mouth, came to a stile which had to be negotiated, he laid the basket on the ground, pushed it gently through a low gap to the other side, and then took a running leap over.'[1]

This kind of behaviour clearly represents the breaking away from the fixity of a precise instinctive response, and we must suppose it to involve a fuller discrimination of features in the situation, and a corresponding plasticity of instinct mechanism rendering possible modification and complication of response. In part we may attribute this growing plasticity to a development in integration, so that it may come about that two or more instinctive tendencies may not only be touched off simultaneously by one situation, but may be so related or arranged as to result in a compromise response,[2] combining features of both specific

---

[1] *The Outline of Science*, sect. vii, vol. I, p. 151.

[2] To borrow again from the chapter referred to in Hobhouse's book : he quotes Romanes, on the authority of Mr. E. L. Layard, as follows : ' I once watched one (i.e. a cobra) which had thrust its head through a narrow aperture and swallowed one (i.e. a toad). With this encumbrance he could not withdraw himself. Finding this, he reluctantly disgorged the precious morsel, which began to move off. This was too much for snake philosophy to bear, and the toad was again seized ; and again, after violent

responses. We may take a simple illustration : the instinct of curiosity once stimulated by a situation leads naturally to the response of approach and investigation. The instinct of escape[1] once stimulated may lead to flight, shamming dead, or concealment. Now many situations are appropriate to the arousal of both these instinctive responses, if the creature concerned is capable of such an experience. In a specifically adjusted creature only one or the other instinct is aroused, which means that only one dominant character in the situation is discriminated for reaction. The biological utility of this for a species which depends entirely on instinctive adaptation is obvious. But the psychological significance of an ability to discriminate two or more significant features in a situation, and to display tendencies to respond to both, cannot be over-estimated : we may indeed trace to that the beginnings of the kind of conscious mental life which, as human, we know introspectively. In the supposed case what we may conceive as happening is the combination of the concealment and the investigation responses, and their fusion in what we might call the cautious approach response. But clearly there is another possibility. A situation may arouse two instincts or tendencies to respond which are entirely incompatible, and cannot in any way coalesce. As both tendencies reach a high intensity they conflict with one another, and the creature falls into a condition of unstable

efforts to escape, was the snake compelled to part with it. This time, however, a lesson had been learnt, and the toad was seized by one leg, withdrawn, and then swallowed in triumph.' Hobhouse comments on this : ' Here there appears a sort of conflict between the impulse to seize, and the necessity of withdrawing the head. The result is a kind of compromise which happens to suit the case well ' (p. 89).

[1] I do not wish to suggest that there is a specific ' escape ' instinct. By an instinct of escape I merely mean one of the group of 'Danger Instincts.' See Rivers, *Instinct and the Unconscious*, ch. vii.

equilibrium until the conflict between the rival tendencies has been successfully determined by inhibition or repression —or until the failure to respond has led to the creature's destruction (this may well be the nature of the ' fascination ' which serpents are said to exercise over their victims). We may note in passing that it is probably at this point of psychological development that the germs of self-feeling and self-consciousness arise—a point to which further reference will be made in the next chapter. It is probable that the back-stroke of a conflict between two or more rival impulses to respond is experienced in the form of affect. That is to say, the condition of mental tension manifests itself in feeling, and the function of feeling may well be, partly at least, to try to end the condition of suspended response, either by a fusion of tendencies, or by the repression of one of the rival tendencies. That, however, is not a point of primary importance to the immediate issue, which is to call attention to the fact of the conflict and co-operation of tendencies at a certain stage of development. But we may now go a step further. Situations in the world actually are far more complex than such partially discriminated ones as can be successfully dealt with through specific responses determined by instincts or other original or compound tendencies : a dog in a picture gallery, as Sir Oliver Lodge remarks, is chiefly ' interested in smells and corners '[1] but the picture gallery as a ' situation ' cannot be fully summed up as an intermixture of interesting smells and attractive corners except for a creature whose endowment does not enable him to discriminate anything further in a situation than that to which

[1] *Reason and Belief*, 1910, p. 100 : ' A dog in a picture gallery, interested in smells and corners, may represent, as in a parable, much of our own attitude to the universe.'

his specific tendencies adjust him. There are situations in the world as much beyond the specific endowment of man as the picture gallery situation is beyond the specific endowment of the dog : but the remarkable and interesting fact that faces us is that in the case of man we know that he has constantly awakened to the vague, and sometimes terrifying, awareness of the fact that he is in the presence of a situation which he is not equipped to deal with on the lines of any existing mechanism. The point at which this awareness arises—wherever in the evolution of mind we may find reason to place it—is obviously of crucial psychological significance, marking the beginning of both intelligence and religion. Where a new response arises, not conditioned by any specific instinctive mechanism, but by some vague and partial discrimination of ' something more ' in the situation than that to which the organism is specifically adapted, we get the breaking through of instinct mechanism as the sole mode of adaptation and response to environment.

I have endeavoured to state the case hitherto in terms as nearly behaviouristic as possible, in order to make clear and vindicate the assertion that it is conceivable (if not probable) that man may have responded to certain phenomena, or situations, with behaviour which we should call worship, or magic, or more generally religion, without having formulated any beliefs, or having become definitely conscious of any ideas. But the facts cannot be at all adequately expressed in these terms. We are actually dealing with the conditions of the dawn of consciousness as we know and understand it : for one of the marks of the transition from man-like ape to ape-like man was the establishment of self-consciousness—which is the only

type of consciousness of which we can frame any clear
picture, and in the total absence of which we should
scarcely classify a claimant to humanity as man. We may,
then, in terms of mind, state the position thus : as consciousness supervenes upon instinct (and the tendencies)—
or as these become more highly integrated and make
possible an awareness which is no longer through instinct
of particular situations, but of the general ends of instincts
as belonging to a system unified under a common life, man
comes into contact with an immense number of features
in his environment in relation to which he is not equipped
by any specific predisposition. He is not under the
immediate urge of a tendency to respond which does not
wait, but fulfils itself ; he has to begin to fabricate the
situation, or features in it, to project something from
himself upon them and endow them in fantasy and
imagination with characteristics which will bring them
within the scope of his active tendencies. The environment is perpetually presenting itself in unfamiliar,
surprising and perplexing aspects ; these features will
have, as it were, a halo of ' beyondness ' or mystery.
But though there is no specific tendency capable of
responding to such a situation, involving the discrimination of a complexity beyond the range of predisposition, the urge to make some response is still there,
being an intrinsic characteristic of any kind of perceptual
experience ; and religion is one of the attempts of man
to overcome the inadequacy of his innate equipment as
he enters into the larger world which is no longer walled
round by specific adaptation mechanisms. We may say,
then, that the religious response is so far from being the
expression of a specific religious tendency or instinct, as

some writers have tried to maintain[1] that it is precisely the outcome of the inadequacy of specific response tendencies. It is man's attempt—or one of his attempts—to supplement the paucity of his original endowment when he discovers himself in a strange world.

We must here note that the failure of innate equipment before a complex situation does not always or necessarily lead to a religious response. Failure may amount to actual break-down as a result of the inter-relation of the tendencies, and lead to collapse, a reaction of which Rivers writes as follows :

> ' This last form of reaction to danger is one which has greatly puzzled biologists. The reaction is usually accompanied by tremors or irregular movements which wholly deprive the reaction of any serviceable character it might possess through the paralysis of movement. . . . We shall take a more natural view of the reaction by collapse if we regard it as a failure of the instinct of self-preservation taking place in animals when instinctive reactions to danger have been so overlaid by reactions of other kinds that, in the presence of excessive or unusual stimuli, the instinctive reactions fail. It is noteworthy that collapse with tremor seems to be especially characterisic of Man in whom all the different modes of reaction to danger found in the animal kingdom are present in some degree, but no one of them so specially developed as to form an immediate and invariable mode of behaviour in the presence of danger.
>
> There is evidence also that collapse and tremor occur especially when there is frustration of an instinctive reaction. Thus, Brehm describes a motionless state, with starting eyes and tongues

[1] See footnote to p. 15 above. Cf. also Rudolf Otto, *The Idea of the Holy*, 1923. With the general attitude of this book the present volume is largely in harmony, but there is this fundamental point of difference, that underlying Otto's treatment throughout is the assertion that what he calls the ' " numinous " state of mind ' is ' perfectly *sui generis* and irreducible to any other.' (p. 7). This seems to me to be equivalent to the admission that no further psychological account can be given of religion than the affirmation that it is the ' numinous ' state of mind, and in a derived sense, all expressions to which this state of mind leads. The purpose of the present inquiry is to try to shew that what Otto calls the ' numinous ' state of mind can be traced back to definite psychological conditions. Otto's basis is thus essentially similar to that of those who postulate a specific religious instinct. See also p. 63, *The Idea of the Holy*. Further : see appendix ii, p. 224, below.

hanging out of their mouths, in seals which had been surprised in their favourite place of repose and cut off from their usual access to the sea. Again, as an example in Man, Mosso observed collapse with violent tremor in a youthful brigand condemned to summary execution. Emitting a shrill cry, the boy turned to flee and rushing against a wall, writhed and scratched against it as if trying to force a way through. Baffled in his attempt to escape, he at last sank to the ground like a log and trembled as Mosso had never seen another tremble, as " though the muscles had been turned to a jelly shaken in all directions." '.[1]

Now this type of reaction is obviously not religious, although it comes, as Rivers says, under the formula of the failure of instinct. But short of a genuine reaction by collapse, which really represents the overwhelming and destruction of the organism by its environment, we have numerous instances of what may be called *reaction by withdrawal :* the most obvious of which is the very familiar response of falling asleep, and of which further instances are afforded in abundance in the psychoses and psycho-neuroses. While the collapse reaction is only one stage short of the actual destruction of the organism, and will almost inevitably lead to that end, the withdrawal reaction represents what may be called the temporary defeat of the organism in its normal functioning. It is the result of the frustration of the mental equipment, but not, as in the case of collapse, of its elimination. Thus while collapse may be described as the last convulsion of an organism incapable of further response, withdrawal is itself a controlled reaction to the situation—a negative response in itself, it is true, but one which provides the opportunity for effecting a new orientation. And the manner in which we find a new orientation in the course of achievement is, as will be more fully shewn later on, through the liberation of fantasies and images, and

---

[1] *Instinct and the Unconscious,* pp. 55-6.

their projection upon the situation which led to the withdrawal. An illustration of this is afforded in the sleep response, as a result of which the tendencies which are under repression or inhibition during the period of waking consciousness are liable to break out into the most vivid images and fantasies in dreams, and the tendencies discharge themselves, and find partial, or even complete, satisfaction, in manipulation of the images and fantasies, and sometimes in overt behaviour in relation to them, as in the case of sleep walking. A still more definite reaction by withdrawal, followed and possibly accompanied by active fantasy and image work, often reaching the stage of hallucinations, is a well-known fact in psychopathology. Thus August Hoch, in urging the importance of the clinical studies of insanity for the understanding of every-day life, says :

> ' No better psychoses could be chosen for a preliminary effort than benign stupors. Every psychiatrist has seen them, although they are wrongly diagnosed as a rule, and they play no small rôle in the world's history. Euripides represents Orestes as having a stupor which is pictured as accurately as any modern psychiatrist could describe an actual case. St. Paul is chronicled as falling to the ground, being thereafter blind and going without food or drink for three days. While apparently unconscious, he had a religious vision. St. Catherine of Siena had several unquestionable stupors, which are fairly well described. In fact, the mystics in general seem to have had communion with God and the saints most often when they seemed unconscious to bystanders '.[1]

It is not suggested that the reaction by withdrawal is a universal and necessary stage through which the percipient must pass in escaping from the world of relatively specific response adjustment to that of intelligence and religion. The point is that it is a striking instance of the type of pre-

---

[1] *Benign Stupors,* 1921, ch. i.

liminary response which actually is made to a situation which is out of range. But the processes which, accompanying or ensuing upon the withdrawal lead from it to the positive response may take place without there being a complete withdrawal reaction. The situation will then be reacted to not as it would be for the hitherto sufficient dispositions or tendencies of the percipient, but as it becomes under the transformation of fantasy and image modification. Two things may happen as a result of this type of response. 1. The situation may be effectively brought under control ; that is, the fantasy and image work may simply provide such an interpretation of the unfamiliar features of the situation as to bring them successfully within the scope of the operation of the tendencies. That, of course, is simply the process of getting to know the hitherto unknown ; a process of more complicated adaptation made necessary by the inadequacy of the specific tendencies, but resulting in the satisfactory restoration of equilibrium between organism and environment. 2. The situation may remain strange, and the response be an inadequate one so far as objective results are concerned, being largely a response to the subjective elements of the fantasy and image which are projected upon the situation. This is what characterizes religious reactions. The mark of a religious response, according to this view, is that a certain incongruity and disparateness is discriminated, and reacted to not in successful adaptation to the actual elements or features of the situation, but in a partial adaptation (which may appear as withdrawal) which still leaves a state of unstable equilibrium. It is not the mere unfamiliarity or strangeness of the situation which initiates this response. It is the discrimination of something which is and remains beyond the capacity of existing equipment ; and it is this ' beyond ', which is initially a frustration experience, which provides the nucleus for all the fantasy and imaginative formations of religious belief. And here we have the germ of the distinction which has played so important a part in the history of religion—that of the two worlds or orders ; this every-day world, which is not necessarily familiar, but which can be effectively treated even where it is unfamiliar ; and that other region, threatening, astonishing, bizarre, powerful, which breaks in at certain points upon this one, in relation to which the existing modes of normal response are utterly inadequate, and remain so.

It is generally agreed among modern writers on this subject that religion cannot be considered in isolation from social life, since it is a social phenomenon. While this is true, there are certain facts which must never be lost sight of by the psychologist, and in particular this : that the group, though probably a much more homogeneous unit in primitive times than now, is and was never a psychological unit in the same sense that the individual is ; and consequently that which is to be established, handed down through custom and by tradition and expressed in a social institution must have its solid background in personal responses. The nature of these personal responses is, of course, largely what it is because of man's inter-relations with his fellows, but a social response which is to link one individual in a common life with others is none the less individual—it is the response of an individual who is urged from within to behave in this particular fashion. It is in this sense that the response to ' beyondness ' is proposed as the germ of all religious behaviour and experience.

That such personal responses cannot be said to be ' religious ' in the rather specific sense that is often adopted in modern speech is of course admitted.   It is only after they have profoundly affected the group life, and become inwrought into the texture of social behaviour and custom that we learn to distinguish their results as religious.   But this sort of difficulty is inherent in the whole story of evolution and its interpretation.   An amœba is not a man ; but the evolutionist tries to trace a thread of continuity all the way through.   A reaction by withdrawal to a situation in which ' beyondness ' is discriminated is not religion in the same sense as Christianity or Buddhism is religion[1] but it is still possible to trace a thread of continuity from the one to the other, and to discern the continued operation of the same fundamental mechanisms.   We can conceive the experienced inadequacy of equipment before a more complex discrimination as the point of departure for what we know as religious development.   Hitherto man (or the ancestor of man, if we discover reason to place this awakening at the period of man's emergence, and regard it as a proprium of humanity) lived in one world, a normal ordinary world, presenting no problems save those which could be solved by the operation of the various tendencies with which he was endowed, or those which arose through conflict, co-operation and fusion under the spur of experience.   In terms of the Genesis myth of the Bible, this was the era previous to the Fall of Man.   But now something awakens in man—for we do not suppose that it was the environment that underwent radical change—which puts him in touch for the first time with problems which do not

---

[1] Though it may be noted that St. Paul's reaction on the Damascus road had a good deal to do with the foundation of Christianity.

carry with them their own solution, situations which baffle his predispositions, and thus the way is open for going wrong. The fall of man from infallibility—or innocence— is in fact the dawn of self-consciousness, and of religion.

We may, then, tentatively regard religion as being essentially an attitude determined by the discrimination of an element of ' utterly-beyondness ', brought about by a mental development which is able to appreciate the existence of more in the world than that to which existing endowment effects adequate adjustment. This mark is no less characteristic of primitive religious phenomena than it is of the most advanced. Amid its almost infinitely diverse modes of specific development in belief and practice the religious attitude never outgrows this fundamental characteristic, and nothing that is without it can intelligibly be called religious.

II

THE MECHANISM OF THE RELIGIOUS RESPONSE

THE conclusion reached in the last chapter was that religious behaviour originates in the discrimination of a situation in relation to which existing equipment, in the form of original or acquired tendencies, is inadequate, and may be said to break down. But, as was shewn, this is the source of more than *religious* behaviour : it may be regarded as the starting point of all self-conscious orientation to the world. For what happens is the initiation of fantasies and images around the situation which has the ' beyond ' character, and these are projected upon the situation in two main ways : (1) a projection which employs the fantasy and image as means through which practical control is gained, and (2) a projection which is in the nature of a partial substitution, the situation not being actually or fully brought under control, and thus the fantastic or imaginal compound is itself responded to in place of the situation. Thus the new response which arises is of a composite character, consisting of (i) fantasy and image work ; (ii) overt action in relation to the situation as affected by this work. Under ii there are two types : (a) the fantasy and image work brings the situation under practical control, and the organism is now in a position to deal with it effectively : and this means that the unfamiliar is now incorporated, by the aid of thought, in the system of that universe to which there is adequate practical adaptation, and (b) the situation remains in actuality out of range even after fantasy and image work, and consequently it is mainly to the fantasy and image that the overt response takes place. The difference is that in the case of (a) the new and strange is successfully assimilated to the old, the customary, the every-day, while in the case of (b) there remains an element of thwarting and baffling which withstands the effort to reduce the situation to familiar simplicity. Here we have the roots of two of the great activities of the human spirit : knowledge, and faith. Knowledge means that the new is fitted into what may be called practical categories—the reduction of fresh and strange situations to elements which can all be successfully and adequately dealt with in action or brought under control. Faith involves the recognition of a persisting element in the situation which eludes control by the functioning of any existing tendencies, and which can only be dealt with on analogy and through fantasy and imagination.[1] This distinction between knowledge and faith could in the nature of things only have come about very gradually, and indeed is by no means firmly established or clearly recognized among modern people. Under primitive con-

---

[1] This seems to me to be implied in much that Inge says about Faith in his volume already referred to. The following are typical statements : ' Faith, then, " transcends experience " ; it appears as a constructive activity. It employs the imagination to fill out what is wanting in experience. Faith endeavours to find harmony in apparent discord, and to anticipate the workings of the divine purpose.' (p. 53) ' Would Faith be Faith if it were not unrealized ? Faith is the felt unity of unreduced opposites. . . . The certainty that all contradictions are reconciled in the eternal world is ours ; but the *how* is mainly hidden from us. Meanwhile, as might be expected while we are feeling our way, there is a borderland of half-beliefs, half-fancies, promptings from our subconscious life, anticipations of later developments. These vague intimations are neither to be rejected nor superstitiously obeyed, but studied and analysed, and above all brought to the test of action, till they yield something definite.' (pp. 235-7) As we have seen, this faith attitude is treated by Inge as the outcome of an instinct ; here it is treated as one of the outcomes of the frustration of instinct equipment.

ditions we may conceive that the result of the first awakening to the strange world which is ' over and above ' that to which man as animal had hitherto been adjusted was a general ' religiousness '[1]—that is to say, the reaction to all really novel situations would be of the fantastic and imaginative kind as against the practical. As R. R. Marett expresses it :

' The chariot of progress, of which the will of man is the driver, is drawn by two steeds, namely, Imagination and Reason, harnessed together. Of the pair, Reason is the more sluggish, though serviceable enough for the heavy work. Imagination, full of fire as it is, must always set the pace. So the soul of the late Palæolithic hunter, having already in imagination controlled the useful portion of the animal world, was more than half-way on the road to its domestication. But in so far as he mistook the will for the accomplished deed, he was not getting the value out of his second horse ; or, to drop the metaphor, the scientific reason as yet lay dormant in his soul.'[2]

Anthropologists have, indeed, collected a great deal of evidence to shew that amongst modern ' primitive ' peoples religion is intermingled with the daily life in a fashion which bears out this supposition.[3] The progress of civi-

[1] Dr. J. T. MacCurdy, who has kindly read this and the preceding chapter, criticizes the use of the term ' religion ' at this level of behaviour, on the ground that what we get back, or down, to is a kind of matrix out of which later on develop religion, intelligence, and other specializations. I have, however, endeavoured to make quite clear what is implied in my use of the term at this level in the preceding chapter, especially pages 4-6.

[2] R. R. Marett, *Psychology and Folk-Lore*, 1920, pp. 240-1.

[3] Lévy-Bruhl, *Primitive Mentality*, 1923, p. 32 : ' The primitive makes no distinction between this world and the other, between what is actually present to sense, and what is beyond. He actually dwells with invisible spirits and intangible forces. To him it is these that are the real and actual. His faith is expressed in his most insignificant as well as in his most important acts. It impregnates his whole life and conduct.' Also p. 89 : ' The all-pervading presence of spirits, witchcrafts, and enchantments ever threatening in the background, the dead so closely connected with the life of the living—this ensemble of representations is an inexhaustible source of emotions to the primitive, and it is to this that his mental activity owes its characteristic features.'
Also W. H. R. Rivers, *Medicine, Magic and Religion*, 1924, p. 49 : ' The religious character of the medical art among such peoples is only one example of the way in which religion and the religious attitude permeate every part of their social life. Religion among such people is not a matter for one day in the week, but influences every act of their daily lives.'

lization has been very largely, in this particular, a matter of releasing territory from the symbolic imagery of faith, and incorporating it in the kingdom of experimental knowledge. It is curious and interesting to reflect, in this connection, that in the period of the ' conflict ' between religion and science many religious apologists attempted to safeguard religion by insisting on ' reserved areas ' in which free inquiry must be prohibited, the tacit assumption being that faith can only survive in the interstices of knowledge—and the ' faithful ' feared that science was too rapidly advancing over areas which had hitherto been in darkness or the twilight of ignorance. This attitude again displays the characteristic already stressed as original in religion, the response, namely, to something outside the range of practical control. The fear of the theologians that there would cease to be any awareness of a ' beyond ' element in consequence of the growth of science, and therefore no place left for the emotional and imaginative reactions of religion, was a curious instance of unnecessary panic. So far from diminishing the extent or immensity of the possible discrimination of the ' beyond ', the progress of science has tended to increase it, and to bring it back again into the most ordinary and common-place situations.[1]

[1] John Fiske, *The Idea of God*, in the course of chapter vii on ' Conflict between the Two Ideas, commonly misunderstood as a Conflict between Religion and Science,' says (p. 107) ' . . . as scientific generalization has steadily extended the region of natural law, the region which theology has assigned to divine action has steadily diminished. Every discovery in science has stripped off territory from the latter province and added it to the former. Every such discovery has accordingly been promulgated and established in the teeth of bitter and violent opposition on the part of theologians.' But that the growth of science has rather enlarged and glorified the area of the theologian is cogently argued by James Martineau in the first chapter of *The Seat of Authority in Religion :* ' A tissue of intellectual order infinitely wide, a history of ascending growth immeasurably prolonged, surely open to the human mind which can read them both, everything that can be asked for a spectacle entirely divine.' (p. 17) The following passage from Starbuck, *The Psychology of Religion*, is also relevant

It has already been maintained that the method of defining religion in terms of a supposed distinction made by the primitive mind between the ' natural ' and the ' supernatural ' is psychologically inaccurate.[1] As an instance of this inaccurate formulation I may cite Westermarck's assertion :

> ' Men distinguish between two classes of phenomena—" natural " and " supernatural ", between phenomena which they are familiar with, and, in consequence, ascribe to " natural causes ", and other phenomena which seem to them unfamiliar, mysterious, and are therefore supposed to spring from causes of a " supernatural " character '.[2]

What men learn to discriminate is that in certain situations they are being presented with a challenge for which they are not prepared, and the classification of such situations, or elements in them, as supernatural, is a matter of relatively recent achievement of thought. This general point of view is shared by the Sociological School, as represented by Durkheim. He contends that all definitions of religion based upon (i) the idea of the supernatural, or (ii) the idea of divinities or gods, are inadequate—a view with which I am in entire agreement But he goes on to construct a

here : ' Where,' he asks on p. 10, ' is there room for Beauty, or for God, in a world whose parts are all labelled, and all of whose workings are understood ? Such a feeling grows out of a mistaken notion of what science can do. Science really gives a final explanation of nothing whatever. All it can do is to bring a little coherency and constancy into the midst of that which is constantly flowing, to explore a little into the ever-enlarging region of the unknown. In applying the methods of science to the study of religion, most of it will always remain out of our grasp. We shall have to content ourselves by working around the outskirts, making an inroad here and there, feeling our way where clear paths fail, until we are able to say of the religious sense, as of every other field we try to explore, we understand it, *because there are bits of it which satisfy the demands of our intelligence sufficiently to give the feel of knowledge by producing steadfastness in our emotional attitudes.* . . . The end of our study is not to resolve the mystery of religion, but to bring enough of it into orderliness that its facts may appeal to our understanding.'

[1] See above, pp. 10, 11.

[2] E. Westermarck, *The Origin and Development of the Moral Ideas*, 1906, vol. ii, p. 582.

definition on the basis of a classification of all things into
the profane and the sacred :

> ' A religion is a unified system of beliefs and practices relative
> to sacred things, that is to say, things set apart and forbidden—
> beliefs and practices which unite into one single moral community
> called a Church, all those who adhere to them '.[1]

But obviously before it can give us any information to say
that religion deals with the sacred, we must have some
criterion by which to judge what it is : the difficulty being,
as we have seen, that practically any object may be
regarded as sacred.   Durkheim offers no real explanation
of this, but seems to take the fact of the distinction as
ultimate, precisely as the distinction between natural
and supernatural is treated by others.   He says :

> ' . . . if a purely hierarchic distinction is a criterion at once too
> general and too imprecise, there is nothing left with which to
> characterize the sacred in its relation to the profane, except their
> heterogeneity. However, this heterogeneity is sufficient to
> characterize this classification of things and to distinguish it
> from all others because it is very particular : *it is absolute.*   In all
> the history of human thought there exists no other example of
> two categories of things so profoundly differentiated or so radically
> opposed to one another '.[2]

Now this may be true—probably is—but it is purely
descriptive, and in no sense explanatory ; it is difficult to
see what difference is made by treating ' sacred-profane '
as ultimate, and treating ' natural-supernatural ' in the
same way.   Unless there are certain objects which have the
character of sacredness as a definite mark which can be
appreciated and responded to, how do they come to be
treated as ' sacred ' at all ?   And the fact that what are
actually held to be sacred objects differs all over the world

[1] *The Elementary Forms of the Religious Life,* by Emile Durkheim, tr.
J. W. Swain, p. 47.
[2] *Op. cit.,* p. 38.

and at various times puts the theory of objective sacredness out of court. Sacredness is projected upon objects, not discriminated in them. Durkheim seems to admit this also :

> ' . . . religious beliefs are only one particular case of a very general law. Our whole social environment seems to us to be filled with forces which really exist only in our own minds. We know what the flag is for the soldier ; in itself, it is only a piece of cloth. . . . Yet the powers which are thus conferred, though purely ideal, act as though they were real ; they determine the conduct of men with the same degree of necessity as physical forces '.[1]

But he does not seem to realize that in that case we need to know how the fundamental distinction comes to be fabricated by the mind. He is content, apparently, to suppose that ' sacred-profane ' is a sort of category of the understanding, which may be variously applied but which must be taken for granted as an original mechanism.

> ' How so ever much the forms of the contrast may vary, the fact of the contrast is universal '.[2]

But this is epistemological rather than psychological, and does not help us to understand what it is that determines the classification of particular phenomena as sacred or profane respectively. The assumption of a mental category impelling towards a universal dichotomy, with the insistence that, wherever the line is drawn, it must be drawn somewhere, leaves us in the air. The approach here proposed is more objective and definitely psychological. It does not postulate, in the first instance, a belief or a quite vague and general mental category, but seeks to give an account of psychological orientation in terms of actual behaviour trends. Belief does not constitute the sacred thing. The

---

[1] *Op. cit.*, pp. 227-8.   [2] *Op. cit.*, p. 39.

experienced inadequacy of psychological equipment, leading to fantasy, together with the real nature of the situation in its relation to the possibility of practical control, gives its sacred or religious character. Thus the sacred ever continues to elude domestication by the methods of ordinary practice and knowledge along the line of the existing original and acquired tendencies. What the sacred is will therefore inevitably vary in different places and times, owing to the co-operation of a large number of factors.

We have still, however, to attempt to give some more definite and precise account of the way in which the religious response comes to be established on the basis of the breaking through of hereditary and acquired tendencies to respond. Mere inadequacy is a negative idea, of which the result might well be simple collapse. In religion, however, we get a very positive, and increasingly complex, set of responses. Assuming that the thesis already advanced is correct—namely that the object to which response is made is that which is discriminated as ' beyond ' the range of existing adaptation—can any account be given of the fact of there being a response at all ? The suggestion made is that the nature of the religious response is peculiar in as much as it does not arise from the ordinary or usual functioning of the tendencies.[1] Must we assume, then, that there was another ' tendency ' asleep, as it were, in the psychic structure of the responder, which only awakened on the call of the newly discriminated situation ? That

[1] The distinction must be borne in mind between what may be called ' first-hand ' and ' second-hand ' religious responses. Once religion is established, with its beliefs and practices, there is inevitably a large measure of ' second-hand ' religious response, conditioned by acceptance on the part of the group of what is authoritatively suggested by the group leaders and elders together with social tradition in general. In the context of this chapter it is ' first-hand ' responses which are to be understood. See also *Varieties of Religious Experience*, p. 6.

would be to reduce the theory of ' tendencies ' to absurdity
—it would be a flagrant instance of their production *ad hoc*
to ' account ' for an otherwise unaccountable phenomenon.
Is the new response, then, nothing more than a compound
of existing tendencies, new only that it involves a fresh
balance among them in relation to the situation ? But we
have already seen that this process appears to be carried
out among the animals ; it comes under the general fact
of the ' plasticity ' of instincts. Plasticity makes for better
adaptation to situations whose features are more discriminated than at the level of ' fixed ' instincts or chain-
reflexes, but it does not provide us with anything which
can be called specifically religious.

It has already been pointed out in the previous chapter
that the process of life and development defeats the method
of analytic reconstruction. Analysis is inevitably something like dissection : it deals with the dead body rather
than the living organism. But there are stages of development in which we simply have to recognize and record the
fact of an established difference. At a certain stage in
mental evolution we find an animal capable of discriminating a complexity in its environment which successfully
challenges it to new forms of activity. We do not know
why : we can only try to give some account of the conditions which appear to be present. Now chief among
these conditions is the factor, repeatedly referred to, but
not yet brought into the forefront of the discussion, of the
new power of discrimination. Discrimination may be
regarded as hitherto a function of the organism which does
not require any hypothesis of subjective awareness. There
is a certain ' pre-established harmony ' between situation
and equipment, and the organism responds through its

appropriate mechanisms because the mechanisms are 'touched off' by the situation. This is no imaginary picture : but simply a description of a great part of the behaviour of ordinary people in every-day life. To take an instance from recent personal observation : My wife and I were playing golf, and in driving off from one tee I badly sliced the ball, and drove it low and hard straight in the direction of the ladies' tee, on which she was standing. I had no time to warn her, but fortunately she was watching. I distinctly saw her bend inward with a rapid movement, which just allowed the ball to pass without striking her. Immediately afterwards she said : ' That was a near thing, and I was absolutely paralysed ; I could not move a muscle.' She was entirely unconscious of having made precisely the necessary and adequate adaptive response to the situation which saved her from what would have been, in all proba-bility, serious hurt. Here, then, is a case of discrimination and adjustment on the level of existing tendencies, with no ' overflow ' discrimination of features which were beyond the scope of such tendencies. The problem here is : What happens, or may be conceived to happen, when the situation not only contains elements in relation to which there is no predisposition for response, but where such elements are actually discriminated ?

A great deal depends upon the extent to which the situation is discriminated as *novel*—as being quite beyond the existing capacity for response. If it is only a novel element in a situation which in its main features conforms to predispositions to behaviour, there may be nothing more than hesitation, followed by a surrender to the urge of a tendency to respond resulting from the strife or co-operation of existing tendencies, in which case the overflow of discrimination is treated as irrelevant, i.e. inhibited or repressed. But it will be otherwise if the situation is one in which the discrimination of unprepared for elements defeats all existing mechanisms of response. Hesitation will then become one of the following : (i) petrification, or collapse ; (ii) a reaction of 'withdrawal' — temporary external inactivity, probably accompanied by intense affect ; (iii) an integration of the percipient capacities, which will devise a new response, bearing possibly little relation to the actualities of the situation, but one which will have the effect of relieving the unbearable tension of an 'impossible' situation. Nor, indeed, are the alternatives (ii) and (iii) mutually exclusive. Withdrawal may be the condition most favourable for such a fabrication of the situation as will make some kind of response possible. And in the first instance this fabrication is itself the new response —or the major part of it, for it removes the inhibition which had been placed upon the total activities by so treating, disguising or interpreting the baffling situation as to bring it into some relation with the existing psychic and motor mechanisms. In other words, equipment not being adequately adjusted to the situation, the situation is taken in hand and fantastically or imaginatively adjusted to equipment.

In some such way as this we must conceive the beginnings of the process of thinking. It may be observed that this view of the primitive nature of fantasy thinking has been expounded at considerable length from the psycho-analytic point of view. Thus Jung distinguishes

' . . . two forms of thinking—*directed thinking* and *dream or phantasy thinking*. The first, working for communication with speech elements, is troublesome and exhausting ; the latter, on the contrary, goes on without trouble, working spontaneously, so to speak, with reminiscences. The first creates innovations, adaptations, imitates reality and seeks to act upon it. The latter, on the contrary, turns away from reality, sets free subjective wishes, and is, in regard to adaptation, wholly unproductive.'

This latter form of thinking, he goes on to point out, is characteristic of antiquity, of modern primitive peoples, and children—and by no means absent in modern civilized man :

'We know, from our own experience, this state of mind. It is an infantile stage. To a child the moon is a man, or a face, or a shepherd of the stars. . . . We know, too, that lower races, like the negroes, look upon the locomotive as an animal, and call the drawers of the table the child of the table '.[1]

'All this experience suggests to us that we draw a parallel between the phantastical, mythological thinking of antiquity and the similar thinking of children, between the lower human races and dreams. This train of thought is not a strange one for us, but quite familiar through our knowledge of comparative anatomy and the history of development, which shows us how the structure and function of the human body are the results of a series of embryonic changes which correspond to similar changes in the history of the race. Therefore, the supposition is justified that ontogenesis corresponds in psychology to phylogenesis. Consequently, it would be true, as well, that the state of infantile thinking in the child's psychic life, as well as in dreams, is nothing but a re-echo of the pre-historic and the ancient.'[2]

This leads directly to the very important distinction between the two processes of imaginative interpretation on the one hand, and fantastic distortion on the other. It may be asserted at once that there is no difference between these processes in regard to origin, though obviously the distinction is one of vital importance in the course of development. The first play of fantasy upon a situation which has led to a withdrawal reaction, or has proved to be beyond the scope of immediate response, is inevitably both

[1] C. G. Jung, *Psychology of the Unconscious*, 1919, pp. 22, 26.
[2] *Op. cit.*, pp. 27-8.

interpretation and distortion. In so far as the fantasy succeeds in bringing man and the situation into relation of a practical kind, the interpretative function is predominant ; but in so far as fantasy merely provides a substitute for a real facing of the situation, distortion is predominant, and the result is the fantastic flight from reality—the final outcome of which in modern life is such a psychosis as dementia præcox.[1]

Does it follow, then, that the primitive religious responses, so obviously arising from the fantastic distortion of situations which are beyond the functioning of hitherto adequate tendencies, are in fact nothing but the ravings of incipient insanity—or, to put it in somewhat less drastic terms, do they merely ' set free subjective wishes ' and are they ' in regard to adaptation wholly unproductive ' ? This, no doubt, would be accepted by those who discover in religion nothing but a form of escape from reality—the invention of a wish-fulfilment which the actual nature of reality sternly withholds. It was this view, no doubt, that Canon B. H. Streeter had in mind in giving his paper, read before the Seventh International Congress of Psychology at Oxford the title—' Is Religion a Psycho-neurosis ? ' He then said :

' The hypothesis has been put forward by certain students of psychology, that man's idea of God is . . . a " projection " upon

[1] Dr. J. T. MacCurdy, in his book, *The Psychology of Emotion, Morbid and Normal*, 1925, speaking of the ' stolid, deteriorated dementia præcox patient ' says (part xi, p. 555) ''he does not sublimate his instinct motivations, they remain at an infantile level and therefore do not assume a form that has any reference to the actual environment ; they are indulged in fantasy. This is possible because the whole personality is changed and with it the function of consciousness, which has now different standards of reality. This altered consciousness does not discriminate between the real and the imaginary, so that outlet, adequate from a perverted standpoint, is obtainable in images for instinct processes that normally would imply action. Real behaviour and imaginal behaviour have become identical.'

the Universe of that passionate need for a Parent's protection which he felt so often when a helpless frightened child, continued or revived under the stress and strain of later life—in other words, that Religion is essentially a Psycho-neurosis.'[1]

It may be admitted at once that if we found a reasonably intelligent modern person trying to adjust himself to the conditions of present day social life by recourse to sympathetic magic, or imitative magic, we should be inclined to diagnose mental aberration. But the reason for this is obvious, and does not mean that we pass the same judgment upon the Bantu or Melanesian magician ; in the course of human experience there has been built up a system of practical knowledge concerning the nature of reality which is commonly mediated to every individual born into the community. That system of knowledge is itself largely dependent upon the successful fantasy thinking

[1] Seventh International Congress of Psychology, *Proceedings and Papers*, pp. 147-57. Also J. T. MacCurdy, in the book referred to on the last page, raises this very question, in connection with a discussion of certain epileptic characteristics. He says (p. 562, ' . . . are we therefore to conclude that the more genuine religion is, the more is it a product of mental disease ? Not at all. The mystical experience and the epileptic's translation are equally unusual, and, in that sense, equally pathological. So then, is genius. Pedestrian creatures regard originality and morbidity with equal distrust. Ordinary people have two ways of judging reality, by sense and feeling. The sense of reality is, essentially, the judgment of the group in which one lives, which is exercised individually in a purely intellectual way. . .

' Under these circumstances, as psychologists, there seems to be only one way of gauging truth and that is the pragmatic method. The mystical experience is, in itself, neither the mark of disease nor of genius ; it is a proof neither of the reality nor of the unreality of the unseen. But, if it affects the subsequent life of the subject it has validity commensurate with the magnitude and quality of the change. This may be in the direction of insanity or of social usefulness. To a certain extent this direction may be predicted by the route followed in moving towards the goal of identification. " To travel hopefully is better than to arrive, and the true success is to labour." One should note that, while the epileptic embraces the Universe *within himself*, the mystic seeks to *melt himself* into the Divine. Both attain the same conviction, that of all-oneness ; both, too, may enjoy the same affect of supreme reality. But one, in losing his life has found it ; the other, in saving his life is losing his only world.' (p. 563)

Further reference is made to the psycho-pathological interpretation of religion in chapter vii, p. 186 below.

carried on by our ancestors, and indeed, not only our ancestors, but by our contemporaries also, for fantasy thinking always goes on hand in hand with the more recently developed ' directed thinking ' and remains an effective partner in all mental work, whether scientific, philosophical or religious.[1] But the person to whom the racial tradition and experience is available who turns from it and regresses to a primitive fantasy response is on the way to insanity—or at least to psycho-neurosis. And short of such pathological regression we may observe that there are at least two types of religion in the modern world, the one characterized by the predominance of the principle of imaginative interpretation, the other by the principle of emotional and fantastic satisfaction.[2] The former might be called ethico-rational, the latter æstheticoemotional. If either of these characteristics is carried to its extreme we pass out of the realm of religion altogether, in the one case into naturalistic ethics, and in the other into a flight from reality which is neurotic and may even be psychotic. The nature of the religious response, whether in its most primitive or most advanced manifestation, is that while it involves a projection of fantasy upon reality, it never completely substitutes the fantasy as subjective product for the reality, but uses it as a means of establishing some sort of contact with it—just as it never accepts reality without some measure of interpretation contributed by the work of the imagination.

From the course of the discussion so far it will have become evident that in attempting to dig down to the roots

---

[1] See, e.g., J. T. MacCurdy, *Instincts and Images*, p. 235, and pp. 244-8.
[2] For a brief discussion of this see my *Psychological Studies of Religious Questions*, 1924, chap. ix.

of the religious response we find them inextricably entangled with the roots of a great deal else in the mental life. To become capable of the discrimination in a situation of features which, while they baffle, yet effectively challenge to a fresh form of adaptation, is the source of a great deal more than religion ; being in fact, as already asserted, the starting point for all consciously intelligent adaptation to environment.[1] And it is quite possible, if not probable, that in essentials this experience is pre-human.[2] Already, however, the distinguishing mark of the religious as against the intelligent response has been fore-shadowed. It differs in the effect it has upon the situation. Where the projection of fantasy or image enables the agent fully to meet the requirements of the situation, and leaves no unresolved problem—that is, where the fantasy or image work supplies an interpretation which fits all the facts of the situation as they affect the agent—the response is an intelligent one, without the marks of religion. But where the fantasy or image work only succeeds in making possible a response to part of the situation, where the agent is still

[1] On this point the following quotations from Starbuck (*op. cit.*) are relevant : ' The years at which conversions really begin (9 or 10 for boys and 11 for girls) coincide fairly with the years at which Dr. Hancock in his experimental tests found a sudden increment in children's ability to reason. . . . Although the same mental processes are not involved in reasoning and in religious awakenings, Dr. Hancock's tests probably indicate a mental capacity which is a necessary condition for attaining spiritual insight.' (p. 35) This is entirely what we should expect if the religious and the reasoning life are both the result of a discrimination of what is over and above the capacities hitherto organized in the form of tendencies to respond. Again : ' *The first two rises in the curves for conversion seem, then, from the psychological standpoint, to correspond to the decline of the sensory elements in consciousness, and the birth of rational insight.*' (p. 37) And : ' Religious awakening is by no means a unique experience, but falls in with the recognized facts of mental assimilation. The instances are numerous in solving problems, making inventions, reaching scientific conclusions, and the like, of persons *feeling after* an idea with unrest and perplexity until the result is finally presented to clear consciousness ready-made.' (p. 110)
[2] See, e.g., Hobhouse, *Mind in Evolution*, chaps. x-xiii.

affected by elements which remain unaccounted for, out
of range, in relation to which fantasy and image are only
in the nature of symbolic representation—we get the
characteristic religious response. But does this account
for subjective religiousness ? It will probably be admitted
as an objective characteristic : but we can hardly suppose
that primitive man, in making a response to a novel
situation, is aware, as we are, that he is responding intelligently, or responding religiously—he will make either
response, probably, with the same freedom from self
consciousness. That is only to say again what has already
been admitted, that what are strictly religious responses
only become differentiated from a kind of matrix which
contains much more, in the course of development. Nevertheless, we must suppose that there is some difference in
experience which is capable of becoming the mark distinguishing the religious from the workaday type of
response for the subject himself. That mark we are
justified in claiming is to be found in affect. The response
which fully meets the immediate requirements of the
situation may be accompanied by affect, but it is affect
which will find adequate discharge in the activity. The
other type of response, which may seem quite as satisfactory, so far as there is any judgment present in the case,
nevertheless is characterized by affect which is not fully
discharged in the response. Consequently the primitive
would not say, ' I am responding religiously ', but it would
feel different to respond religiously from what it would to
respond practically, and when introspection begins this
feeling is recognized as the sign of the presence in the
situation of unaccountable forces—as the preliminary
conscious response to ' beyondness '. Let me offer, by

way of illustration, an analysis of the factors involved in two situations of this kind : (1) I am disturbed in the middle of the night in my bedroom by an unusual and mysterious tapping noise, and (2) man faced by a shortage of rain, without which ' vegetation withers, animals and men languish and die '.[1]

(1) I happened to record, not long after the event, an instance of disturbance by an unusual noise, and I here quote the words in which I made the record :

' I remember an instance which puzzled me much at the time—a strange tapping sound which I was certain was in the room and not outside, and there was nothing obvious to account for it. It was so insistent and so inexplicable that it disturbed me, and I felt I must solve the problem. Now this is quite similar to the position of the scientific investigator ; he has some fact of observation, and he wants to give an account of it, and what he does in a much more detailed and minute way, I set out to do—i.e., to try experiments. The whole situation to be investigated is the bedroom, with the usual furniture and conditions, plus an apparently alien additional circumstance, the noise. Not being, shall I say, a convinced believer in the likelihood of this tapping being a means of supernatural communication, I assumed it must be due to a natural cause, and that therefore there must be some specific circumstance present in the room which ordinarily is not there. How am I to discover what this is ? Simply by a process of careful abstraction—a simplification of the conditions which are too many and confused as they stand for me to recognize the strange element. So what I did was to say : '' What would happen if I removed my watch, which is hanging on the back of the bed ?—maybe I am shaking the bed, and that causes the chain to swing and tap the wood. I shall find out only by abstracting that feature from the whole situation ''. I did so, and the noise continued. I went on then varying details in the whole situation with no effect, till at last I happened to move a hot water bottle which I had long since put out of bed. The noise stopped. I concluded that it was the source of the noise, and a further brief investigation led to the discovery that there was some slight leakage at the cork which produced the peculiar gurgling noise.'

Now unless we reduce the theory of tendencies to absurdity, it is clear that my behaviour in this situation cannot be

[1] Sir J. G. Fraser, *The Golden Bough*, vol. i, p. 247.

accounted for adequately as the outcome of tendencies touched off by features in the external environment. What we have is precisely a case of the temporary baffling of existing tendencies, leading to freshly constructed responses. Curiosity and fear were both baffled, for the situation did not admit of any direct investigation : it was definitely a case in which activity could only effectively be initiated after some kind of imaginative or conceptual interpretation of the situation had taken place. A fleeting image—or thought—of the watch, of a piece of creeper blown by the wind against the window—was projected upon the situation, and response then made to that reconstructed situation. It is of no consequence that in this instance the actual solution was achieved by a perceptual experience which had not been in any way pre-imagined : for that perceptual experience was only possible because responses had been released by imaginative manipulation of the situation. The essential characteristic about this is that the situation was brought quite definitely under practical control : I could cause the noise to cease, or allow it to continue as I pleased, and could reproduce the conditions under which the noise could be again emitted. Thus there was no remainder of thwarted conation, no element left of a 'beyond' character. The whole series of responses, initiated in the same way as a series that might have been, or might have become, religious, was intelligent for precisely this reason. Had the situation entirely baffled me, and continued to do so until I had projected upon it the fantasy or imagination (whether by accepting it from popular belief, or by originating it myself) of a supernatural, or unaccountable entity making the tapping, it would have been of the religious kind. And behind such a projected fantasy there would have been the affect that distinguished a practically inexplicable situation from a religiously explicable one.[1]

(2) In the same way, we cannot assume the existence of a 'religious instinct' or tendency which impels man to respond to a drought situation either by magic or supplications to 'supernatural' powers. I take a single instance from a large number collected and reported by Sir J. G. Frazer :

> 'Amongst the Omaha Indians of North America, when the corn is withering for want of rain, the members of the sacred Buffalo Society fill a large vessel with water and dance four times round it. One of them drinks some of the water and spirts it into the air, making a fine spray in imitation of a mist or drizzling rain. Then he upsets the vessel, spilling the water on the ground ; whereupon the dancers fall down and drink up the water, getting mud all over their faces. Lastly, they squirt the water into the air, making a fine mist. This saves the corn '.[2]

It is not suggested that this fairly complicated ritual is a genuinely primitive response to the drought situation ; but that it is more nearly primitive than the attitude of a modern meteorologist, and it serves to illustrate the presence and functioning of fantasy in relation to a 'beyond'

---

[1] The hold-up of existing tendencies, followed by affect and imagery projected upon the situation, leading to a reconstructed situation which can be practically dealt with, may characterize life at lower levels than human. Dr. J. T. MacCurdy suggests such an interpretation for certain types of dog behaviour, in his paper, *Instincts & Images* (7th Inter. Cong. of Psych., *Papers & Proceedings*, pp. 232-51). Thus on p. 242 : 'When the dog tries to get under the fence and fails, an image arises of getting under at another place. This stimulates movement to the appropriate part. When he arrives there an image arises of his master lifting the wire. In order that this may occur in fact, he whines to attract his master's attention and leads him to the spot. The images, then, set up reactions which facilitate the experiencing of new perceptions or new images and these in turn induce new reactions, until the whole performance is successfully accomplished. Trial and error is thus reduced to a minimum. ' This is an example of true planning and any dog-lover can duplicate such examples chosen from the observation of isolated behaviour on the part of " intelligent " dogs.'

[2] *The Golden Bough*, vol. i, p. 249.

situation. Clearly, what initiates this response is the discrimination of something in the environment which threatens to defeat all the normal efforts of the group to secure corn. It is no longer a mere fact that drought occurs, and that man, in common with other animals, endures what comes, survives or perishes by such specific adjustments to the sequence of drought conditions as he is capable of making, point by point. It is the definite discrimination of a set of conditions to which there is no reply ready in the mental constitution. No fusion or co-operation of tendencies can be supposed automatically to take place where the essential feature of the situation as discriminated is wholly out of relation with any tendency to action. The instinct of nutrition can hardly be endowed with the function of elaborating methods of making rain, at least without the intervention of a new factor. Under its urge man seeks for food, learns to sow seed, dig the earth and so forth, for these things are matters of perceptual learning ; but there are no perceptual data for initiating the behaviour which aims at controlling the rainfall. That can only be explained as the result of fantasy in connection with the ' beyond ' feature, culminating in the projection of imaginal amendment or supplement upon the situation. To this amended or interpreted situation, response becomes possible. We need not suppose as Frazer implies, that there is any clear cut concept concerning the operation of forces which can be controlled : the simple projection of self feeling, or the fantasy of the self, upon the weather situation, would be adequate to remove the barriers to action imposed by the actual inaccessibility of the situation. Imitative ' magic ' would then be one of the most natural responses, though at this stage of

thought there is nothing ' magical ' about it.   It is one of
the most universal laws of psychology, animal or human,
for the gregarious species, that behaviour is contagious.
Example is more eloquent than precept.   The much
discussed and extremely widespread power of suggestion[1]
is in essence the fact that throughout a gregarious group
types of behaviour tend to reproduce themselves.   To
project the fantasy, therefore, upon the weather, or the
rainfall, that it is a self, is to bring it under the operation
of the same influences as those to which other selves are
subject.   Consequently if the important people of the tribe
set about the business of making rain, the rain itself will
hardly be able to help falling ; just as if one member of
a circle yawns, the rest almost invariably follow suit.   This,
of course, is not the only way of influencing selves.   Much
depends upon the social status of the self or selves to be
influenced, and on the nature of the predominant social
relationship forms.[2]   An inferior self may be forced, an
equal self may be persuaded, a superior self may be peti-
tioned ; in the first case the ritual or practice resulting is
commonly called ' magic ', in the third it is commonly
called ' religion ', while in the second it is sometimes one,
sometimes the other : but psychologically the distinction
between magic and religion is irrelevant, for the same
fundamental mechanism is involved equally in both.   But
what, we now go on to ask, is the result of the response to

[1] This, of course, is not the whole story of suggestion, concerning which
there exists a considerable literature.   But it is usually regarded as being
closely related to the gregarious instinct.   Reference may be made to
Rivers, *Instinct and the Unconscious*, Trotter, *Instincts of the Herd in
Peace and War*.   Also art. in British Journal of Medical Psychology on
Suggestion (vol. iii, pt. i, Jan. 1923) by myself.
[2] F. C. Bartlett, *Psychology and Primitive Culture*, 1923, p. 37, distinguishes three : ' The three fundamental relationships are : primitive
comradeship, assertiveness, and submissiveness.'

the fabricated situation ? We are at least in a position to state, on a basis of very high probability, that it cannot have been an infallible means of securing the required result, and yet we are faced by the fact that this type of response actually established itself with astonishing persistence, not merely as a primitive mode, but in the religious practice of all the generations :

> ‘ Such attempts (says Frazer) are by no means confined, as the cultivated reader might imagine, to the naked inhabitants of those sultry lands like Central Australia and some parts of Eastern and Southern Africa, where often for months together the pitiless sun beats down out of a blue and cloudless sky on the parched and gaping earth. They are, or used to be, common enough among outwardly civilized folk in the moister climate of Europe.’[1]

Prayers are included in *The Book of Common Prayer* ‘ For Rain ’ and ‘ For Fair Weather ’, and these, presumably, are still used, and it is probable that the number of petitions offered up for rain or for fine weather in the course of any year in Christian Churches is quite considerable. What is the reason for this, since we may safely assume that success cannot have been the condition leading to the persistence of so curious a response ?[2] The answer is that

[1] Sir J. G. Frazer, *The Golden Bough*, i, p. 247-8.
[2] Cf. Durkheim’s statement of this question, and his answer, *Elementary Forms*, pp. 79-80 : ‘ . . . the conception of the universe given us by religion, especially in its early forms, is too greatly mutilated to lead to temporarily useful practices. Things become nothing less than living and thinking beings, minds or personalities like those which the religious imagination has made into the agents of cosmic phenomena. It is not by conceiving of them under this form or by treating them according to this conception that men could make them work for their ends. It is not by addressing prayers to them, by celebrating them in feasts and sacrifices or by imposing upon themselves fasts and privations, that men can deter them from working harm and oblige them to serve their own designs. Such processes could succeed only very exceptionally and, so to speak, miraculously. If, then, religion’s reason for existence was to give us a conception of the world which would guide us in our relations with it, it was in no condition to fulfil its function, and people would not have been slow to perceive it : failure being infinitely more frequent than successes, would have quickly shown them that they were following a false route, and religion, shaken at each instant by these repeated contradictions, would not have been able to survive.’ The actual reason, according to Durkheim, for the persistence of such responses is that they are conditioned by that

psychologically this sort of response was—and to some modern civilized people still is—successful : it provided an exit from an impossible situation. In giving an interpretation of the situation to which response of any sort could be made, it brought about the relief of psychological tension which resulted from the blocking of the outlets to activity. Thus as soon as man learned to discriminate situations in regard to which no specific adaptations were ready, he had to evolve some means of discharging activity in relation to them if he were to gain a foothold for himself in the wider world that was opening out to him. This was his effort to make himself at home in a new and strange universe. But in this instance, as contrasted with that concerning myself, the fact is that the response was successful psychologically, not materially : it did not objectively relate the situation to human equipment and need. There remained something left over, an element of uncertainty and incalculability, manifest in affect, and that constitutes it religious. Response to a situation by means of imaginative interpretation which, however, does not reduce the situation to

reaction to the social group which he treats as the essence of religion. Thus, p. 225 : ' Its primary object is not to give men a representation of the physical world, for if that were its essential task, we could not understand how it has been able to survive, for, on this side, it is scarcely more than a fabric of errors. Before all, it is a system of ideas with which the individuals represent to themselves the society of which they are members, and the obscure but intimate relations which they have with it. This is its primary function ; and though metaphorical and symbolic, this representation is not unfaithful . . . for it is an eternal truth that outside of us there exists something greater than us (sic), with which we enter into communion.' As against this the following passage from C. G. Jung's *Psychology of the Unconscious*, p. 262, may be quoted, with which the view adopted above is in harmony : ' The religious myth meets us here as one of the greatest and most significant human institutions which, despite misleading symbols, nevertheless gives man assurance and strength, so that he may not be overwhelmed by the monsters of the universe. The symbol, considered from the standpoint of actual truth, is misleading indeed, but it is *psychologically true*, because it was and is the bridge to all the greatest achievements of humanity.'

certainty and calculability and allow the adequate discharge of affect, so that there is always an element of ' beyondness ' and mystery, an unanalyzed remainder, an unresolved problem, is religion.

The objection may be raised to this formulation that while it covers the religious response of a considerable number of modern people, who would definitely trace the religious nature of their ideas or behaviour to the recognition or feeling of a background of uncertainty and mystery,[1] it is surely in striking contrast, or even conflict, with outstanding facts both of modern primitive and historic religion. Regarding this objection, it must suffice here to point out that the facts which at first sight seem to be out of harmony with the theory advanced, are in the main confirmatory evidence. The objection will be based chiefly on the fact that religion, in most of its institutional forms, has been characterized by a dogmatic certitude and oppressive confidence about the nature of ultimate things that has, from time to time, alienated the more independent minds, and that therefore, so far from a recognition of ' beyondness ', religion has been characterized by a most emphatic assurance of full possession of the real secret. But this dogmatic attitude differs profoundly from the attitude of the human mind to knowledge which has been attained by experimental methods, and has been subjected to the processes of verification.[2] It appears much more

---

[1] See appendix iii, p. 231.

[2] W. Trotter states in his *Instincts of the Herd in Peace and in War* that the primary need of the herd as such is for *certitude*, and the appearance of reason is therefore an unwelcome intervention in the course of instinctive certitude. The majority of people have the strongest and most rigid opinions on these subjects about which they know least. ' Nowadays matters of national defence, of politics, of religion are still too important for knowledge, and remain subjects for certitude.' (pp. 34-5) The point is referred to in my *Psychological Studies of Religious Questions*, chap. xiv.

like a defence reaction against uncertainty than the expression of a reasonable conviction.[1] Precisely because religion is an attempt to deal with that which lies beyond man's ordinary equipment, it claims for its formulations an authority and a sanctity altogether above reason. We come here upon the whole question of revelation and its psychology. The strange world that lies beyond the workaday world to which the ordinary person is adjusted cannot be known or responded to unless some kind of relationship is established between it and the human being. The tendency for all established religions, which here depart from the method and vision of the original founders,[2] is to assert that supernatural revelation is the means by which the world beyond communicates itself, that this revelation has been once and for all delivered to the saints—the special caste of priests, or other religious authority—and that any tampering with the substance of revelation, as safeguarded by the special caste or religious organization, will be attended with incalculable pains and penalties. Moreover, even on the part of those who regard themselves as the custodians of the revelation, an essential element of radical uncertainty still persists : the formulations (in creed, ritual or other traditional way) which they have received are not regarded as exhausting the Beyond, which at any moment may break in upon this world in unexpected and incalculable fashion ; these formulations actually give,

[1] Cf. C. G. Jung, *Psychology of the Unconscious*, p. 261 : ' The rule is a great uncertainty among believers, which they drown with fanatical cries among themselves or among others ; moreover, they have religious doubts, moral uncertainty, doubts of their own personality, feelings of guilt and, deepest of all, great fear of the opposite aspect of reality, against which the most highly intelligent people struggle with all their force.'

[2] William James, *The Varieties of Religious Experience*, 1919, on p. 30, says : ' Churches, when once established, live at second-hand upon tradition ; but the *founders* of every church owed their power originally to the fact of their direct personal communion with the divine.'

according to the authoritarian point of view, the utmost concerning the beyond that can be humanly grasped—that portion of the Ultimate the knowledge of which (or rather the faith in which) is essential but adequate for man's safety here and hereafter. The conserving tendencies operate upon such customs and beliefs as have given man a foot-hold in the larger world of the mysterious, and all the weight of social suggestion re-inforces the authority of the successful adaptations to the dangerous and mysterious regions. It is precisely when some overwhelming experience of a reality which is not in any adequate way mediated through dogma and established custom breaks in upon an individual or a group that the reformation of religion takes place, or a new religion is initiated. That is to say, we have once again the operation of the principle laid down as fundamental in the religious response : the ability to discriminate a ' still-beyond ' element. Every fresh impetus in religion is traceable to this fundamental discrimination ; and a recognition of this fact brings into prominence the two contrasted types of religion : (i) the traditional, priestly, mediated—one which depends for its stability very largely on the influence of suggestion and other social factors, and (ii) the heretical, prophetic, immediate—one which is the direct response of personality to the challenge of a Beyond which is experienced at first-hand.

III

A STUDY OF THE RELIGION OF THE WINNEBAGO INDIANS

In making the attempt to determine the character of religion from the psychological point of view we are not solely, or even primarily, concerned with the question of the actual origin of religion. Indeed, in one sense, we are not concerned with that question at all. In last resort the actual origin of religion can only be dealt with under the form of a myth. There are, and in the nature of the case there can be no materials available out of which to construct a historically accurate account of the actual first emergence of religious behaviour. But on the other hand, it must be one of the postulates of psychology in this, as in any other branch, that if we can analyse any complex into simple elements which are not further reducible, these simple elements are basic and fundamental for all manifestations which can legitimately be classified as belonging to the complex in question. Such a complex is religion. If we can analyse in its typical forms a common irreducible element such as the ' beyond ' discrimination—or what Rudolf Otto[1] calls the ' numinous consciousness '—we must assume that whenever and however religion first came into existence, it did so on the basis of this element. It is in that sense that the ' origin ' of religion is treated in these pages. In what follows I propose to try to shew the

---

[1] *The Idea of the Holy*, 1923. See appendix ii, p. 224.

working of this fundamental principle in specific contexts, and to endeavour to demonstrate that in definite historical periods of religious expansion or new outburst, this deepened awareness of the 'utterly beyond,' bringing about the defeat of hitherto adequate modes of adaptive response, and leading to a new personal orientation, has been an invariable and formative characteristic.

Instead of a wide survey of modern primitive religions with a view to selecting here and there illustrative material to support the theory, I propose to follow the lead given by Mr. F. C. Bartlett in his *Psychology and Primitive Culture*, and to make an intensive study of a particular phase of the religious development of a particular tribe. In choosing the Winnebago Indians for this purpose I do so for the following reasons.

(1) Dr. Paul Radin, the author of the detailed monograph on *The Winnebago Tribe* in the Bureau of American Ethnology Series, himself suggested this material, together with his *Sketch of the Peyote Cult of the Winnebago*, in conversation concerning the theory of the religious response here developed, as bearing out and illustrating the thesis.

(2) The material is fully and carefully presented by an expert investigator, who has made an exhaustive study of the social and religious life of this tribe.

(3) Though Mr. Bartlett has made use of part of this material, he has done so mainly for the purpose of a study in the conditions of culture transmission, and not for the purpose of a study of the psychological factors at work in religious development and expansion.

(4) The Winnebago, though not by any means among the most 'primitive' of the tribes whose life and habits have been carefully studied, nevertheless represent an

outlook much simpler and more direct than that of highly developed and civilized religious communities ; and they are shewn in process of adaptation to the searching conditions of a new environment, constituted by the impingement of the civilization of the West. This provides a ' beyond ' situation which affords a particularly valuable opportunity for testing the theory.

The first contact of the Winnebago with white men was in 1634, but unfortunately there is no contemporary record of this event. We learn, however, that about this period the Winnebago appear to have been warlike, treacherous, and cannibalistic. We are not here concerned with the history of their alliances and warfares which, Radin says, were ' the most important events of Winnebago history during the eighteenth century ',[1] but rather with the aspect of life which is admirably represented in the account of the ' coming of the Frenchman Decora among them and his marriage to the daughter of the chief of the tribe '.[2] This account has been preserved by the Decora family, and is, Radin says, ' clearly mixed up with what we believe is an account of the first contact of the Winnebago with the French '.[3]

The account starts with the origin of the Winnebago.

> ' They had no tools to work with at that time. All they had were bows and arrows and a fire-starter. They had no iron, and if they saw a stone that was naturally sharpened in any way, it was considered sacred and they offered tobacco for it. They had tobacco from the beginning. It was their most valued possession '.[3]

The practical nature of religion, a point brought out more

---

[1] *Thirty-seventh Annual Report of the Bureau of American Ethnology*, Washington, Government Printing Office, 1923, p. 58.

[2] *Op. cit.*, p. 65.

[3] *Op. cit.*, the full account occupies pp. 65-9, from which the present summary and excerpts are made.

specifically on p. 278, and at the same time its interpenetration with common life and interest are indicated : they fasted and became holy, offered tobacco to the spirits and gave feasts so that they might become successful in war. An explanation of the religious significance and function of tobacco follows : Earthmaker created man last of all creatures, and feeblest of all—he alone had not control over anything. But finally Earthmaker created a weed with a pleasant odour, and mashing up a leaf of it, shewed how it should be smoked, and gave the spirits a puff of it. This caused them all to long for the control of it, but Earthmaker handed it over to man, because he was so weak.

> ' This weed will be called tobacco. The human beings are the only ones of my creation who are poor. I did not give them anything, so therefore this will be their foremost possession, and from them we will have to obtain it. If a human being gives a pipeful and makes a request we will always grant it.' Thus spoke Earthmaker.

There follows the story of the coming of the French in ships upon the lake. The Winnebago went to meet them with tobacco and deer-skins ; the French fired a salute of guns, whereupon

> ' The Indians said " They are thunderbirds." They had never heard the report of a gun before that time, and that is why they thought they were thunderbirds.'

Actual intercourse was difficult because the French did not know what to do with tobacco, while the Indians were afraid of the axe with which the French chopped wood for them,

> ' because they thought that the ax was holy. Then the French taught the Indians how to use guns, but they held aloof for a long time through fear, thinking that all these things were holy.'

The manner in which the Winnebago overcame their dread of the ' holy ' things is probably well illustrated by the following incident, next recorded in the narrative :

> ' Suddenly a Frenchman saw an old man smoking, and poured water on him. They knew nothing about smoking or tobacco. After a while they got more accustomed to one another.'

We may safely conjecture that it was such a display of ignorance on the part of the French that saved them from being treated, with their guns and axes, as dangerous and ' holy '.   Had they known all about smoking and tobacco, and thus shewn familiarity with the way of the Indians while displaying new and strange things and ways to them, their appearance would almost certainly have been regarded as that of spirits.   But fortunately (?) for the future of trade and general intercourse the French shewed themselves humanly fallible.   To the Winnebago it was an axiom that all the spirits knew about tobacco, and would do almost anything for it.

The narrative then jumps to the marriage of Decora with the daughter of the Winnebago chief.   He lived with the tribe for a while and two sons were born.   The elder he took away with him when he was ' somewhat grown up ', leaving the mother to bring the other son up among the Winnebago.   Later, however, the elder son desired to return and accordingly Decora brought him back, and said :

> ' My sons are men, and they can remain here and grow up among you.   You are to bring them up in your own way and they are to live just as you do.'

The conclusion of the account, dealing with the attitude of the tribe to Decora's sons, and more generally to the white men, merits quotation in full :

' The Indians made them fast. One morning the oldest one got up very early and did not go out fasting. His older uncle, seeing him try to eat some corn, took it away from him, and, taking a piece of charcoal, mashed it, rubbed it over his face, and threw him out of doors. He went out into the wilderness and hid himself in a secret place. Afterwards the people searched for him everywhere, but they could not find him. Then the people told the uncle that he had done wrong in throwing the boy out. The latter was sorry, but there was nothing to be done any more. In reality the uncle was afraid of the boy's father. They looked everywhere but could not find him.

' After a full month the boy came home and brought with him a circle of wood (i.e., a drum). He told the people that this is what he had received in a dream, and that it was not to be used in war ; that it was something with which to obtain life. He said that if a feast was made to it, this feast would be one to Earthmaker, as Earthmaker had blessed him and told him to put his life in the service of the Winnebago.

' From this man they received many benefits. He was called to take the foremost part in everything. They called him the Frenchman, his younger brother being called Tcap 'o'sgaga, White throat. And as they said, so it has always been. A person with French blood has always been the chief. Only they could accomplish anything among the whites. At the present time there is no clan as numerous as the descendants of that family and the object that he said was sacred (the drum) is indeed sacred. It is powerful to the present day. His descendants are the most intelligent of all the people, and they are becoming more intelligent all the time. What they did was the best that could be done. The ways of the white man are the best. This is the way they were brought up.

' This is the end of the history of the Decoras.'

There are several points in this narrative that are illuminating for the study of religious psychology. We meet here with the formulation of the ' holy ' ; we learn that among the Winnebago fasting has a special place among religious acts and is intimately connected with ' holiness ' ; we have a more or less reflective account of man's relation with the spirits and Earthmaker ; and we have the story, probably incorporating an oral tradition, of the first contact with the white man, and a further indication of the attitude of the Winnebago to the element of mystery which surrounded the white man and his habits in the story of Decora's sons, leading up to the outbreak of prophecy.   It will be convenient to study the Winnebago religion under these headings, and in the next chapter to deal with the introduction and development of the Peyote cult.

I : *The Idea of the Holy and Sacred.* ' If they saw a stone that was naturally sharpened in any way it was considered sacred and they offered tobacco for it.'   According to the theory here being advocated the source of the holy or sacred is in the experience of frustration which results from the fuller discrimination of elements in the environment in relation to which there are no existing predispositions.   But we shall not expect to be able to state that every judgment of holiness or sanctity is the direct and immediate outcome of such an experience.   For while a first-hand contact with and recognition of the mysterious is an original element in the determination of the religious response, it does not necessarily continue to operate directly in religion once established as an institution ;   indeed, religion as an established institution is largely a protection to the group against any too direct and immediate contact with aspects of reality which might lead to frustration.[1]   The establishment of a particular religion is really the stamping in of a ' group difference tendency '[2] whose function is to conserve and maintain responses originally determined by the general

---

[1] See below, p. 179 f.

[2] F. C. Bartlett, *Psychology and Primitive Culture*, p. 45. ' . . . as a result, largely, of the operation of the tendencies towards construction and conservation, characteristic institutions arise within a group and are perpetuated.   Such institutions vary in their nature from group to group in accordance with the interplay of the social relationships involved, the specific interests that are aroused, and the nature of the group's external environment.   But once an institution is formed and persists, around it cluster special tendencies having a social reference, and all the appearance of original simplicity.'

factor of the frustration experience together with the more specific factors of particular environment, tradition and social relationship forms. Such a group difference tendency means a habit of reaction which is initiated not merely by the specific elements of mystery which originated the religious response but also by such other objects and situations as come in the course of experience to be associated with them. In other words, religion which has attained institutional status, and gathered around itself definite tendencies to behaviour, assimilates to itself fresh elements of human experience—a characteristic already noted on page 34. To take the instance of the sharpened stones : we can hardly suppose that such objects would be significant enough in themselves, and without a halo of derived associations, to originate the experience of frustration. But once the religious response has been initiated, it is entirely comprehensible that there should be an overflow, and that once man had become educated in the art of seeing more in things around him than those qualities or characteristics of the environment that can readily and immediately be controlled, he would begin to endow many hitherto indifferent things with a halo of fantasy, and to perceive them as therefore mysterious. Naturally sharpened stones, differing from ordinary stones only slightly in objective fact, nevertheless were capable of setting into activity the processes of imaginative and fantastic thinking with the result that the total situation represented by ' these unnatural stones ' together with emotion and imagery, became uncanny—beyond the sphere of customary modes of reaction. The stones represent something more than appears on the surface, which makes itself conscious in the feeling of the uncanny, and gains some kind of vague

interpretation in imagery.   It matters little whether this
something is formulated into the idea of a god, spirit or
demon, or whether the object-together-with-mental-state
is simply felt and reacted to as uncanny ; according as
imaginative work preponderates over purely affective
experience, there will tend to be idea formation.

An interesting feature of the Winnebago religion seems
to be the great extent to which it had become rationalized.
Radin gives a remarkable indication of this in his preliminary description of the religion :

> ' Among the Winnebago religion is definitely connected with
> the preservation of life values.   It is not a phenomenon distinct
> from mundane life, but one of the most important means of
> maintaining social ideals.   What these are can be gleaned from
> practically every prayer ; they are success, happiness, and long
> life.   The vast majority of investigators are often surprised at
> the intense religious life which, among the North American Indians,
> exists side by side with an intense realism and a clear understand-
> ing and appreciation of the materialistic basis of life.   The ex-
> planation, to judge from the Winnebago data, is simple enough.
> The Indian does not interpret life in terms of religion, but religion
> in terms of life.   In other words, he exalts the world around him
> and the multifarious desires and necessities of the day, so that
> they appear to him bathed in a religious thrill.   At least that
> is what the devoutly religious man does and most of the religious
> data presented in this volume emanates from him.   Still, we are
> convinced that for the vast majority of Winnebago, in other words,
> for the intermittently religious, there are many moments in
> life and many actions which are seen through this pleasurable
> religious thrill.'[1]

Now this is not a congenial atmosphere for the ' holy ' or
for religion in its original and fundamental sense.[2]   Derived,

---

[1] 37th Annual Report of the American Bureau of Ethnology, p. 278.

[2] See above, pp. 37-38.   Radin himself calls attention again to the
importance of distinguishing between testimony regarding the feeling
of the religious man, and the intermittently or non-religious man.   The
latter—who generally predominates in any community—may accept the
beliefs and perform the ceremonies of religion with conviction and devotion,
but he is the recipient and participator, not the contributor and originator.
The first-hand religious man develops a keen consciousness of the holy
or sacred, and is likely to find it breaking in upon him not merely through
traditional channels, but in fresh and unexpected ways. *Op. cit.*, p. 177.

or secondary religion, will flourish more conspicuously, and may well be treated as the expression of group tendencies established on the basis of an earlier, ancestral, religious experience. But what we can see in the relatively calm atmosphere of a rationalized religion which has the weight of social authority behind it, is the reference of the judgment of ' holy ' or ' sacred ' to the past. This is very clearly indicated in the mythological elements of Winnebago religion, and in connection with the special rituals of the Medicine Dance and the Clan War Bundle Feasts.[1] In the account summarized above it comes out in the phrase, ' they (i.e., the Winnebago ancestors) fasted and became holy '. It is not so much that there is any definite theory that the past as such is holy, but that whatever comes down from the past is accorded authority and submitted to with obedience as something beyond the right or power of the members of the group to criticize.

Thus in actuality the ' holy ' for the Winnebago appears to have become almost indistinguishable from the success-giving. For there is evidence here that, as amongst the Hebrews at the time of the Job poem, misfortune, disease and other ills are taken as direct indications of unholiness, or what is much the same thing, unauthorized interference with the holy ; while success and prosperity are the overt evidence of holiness. Thus Radin says that the term :

' Wa'ka^n seems exactly equivalent to our word " sacred ". . . . If a Winnebago were to come across some unusually shaped object he might offer tobacco to it, and upon being questioned he would undoubtedly say that the object is wak'a^n. What is it that he means by wak'a^n ? From my experience in the field he simply means that it is " sacred ", and if pressed for a more definite answer he would probably say that it has the power of

[1] Fully described by Radin, *op. cit.*, chapters xiv and xvii.

bestowing blessings upon him—in other words, of acting like a spirit, a waxopᶜi'ni. That is why he offers tobacco to it.'[1]

This value of ' holiness ' or sanctity is well illustrated in the account of J's fasting :·

> ' When I reached the age of puberty my father called me aside and told me to fast. He told me it was his fervent wish that I should begin to fast, so that I might become holy and invincible and invulnerable in war. .'. . He assured me that if I fasted I would really be holy and that nothing on this earth would be able to harm me. I would also live a very long life, he told me. I would be able to treat the sick and cure them. That holy I would be, he told me . . . '[2]

This particular Winnebago, however, ' ate the peyote ', and came to disbelieve in the old ways. The conclusion of his account is none the less interesting :

> ' Indeed, I am holy. If a man is sick I can restore him to health. That is what I used to think. I really (had it been true) should have felt it, for I laboured earnestly and honestly to be a holy person. Yet in spite of all my exertions I was very unfortunate. I had married twice and both my wives and all my children died. Indeed, how could I ever consider myself a holy man, i.e., if I couldn't even cure my own wife and children of what value were my " supernatural powers " ? '[3]

Yet even in this apparently degenerate estimate of the holy and the sacred it is not difficult to discern the survival in the form of tradition of the genuine religious response ; that is to say, the effort to get into effective relations with that something in the total environment which frustrates and eludes man's normal capacities. The intensity of the emotional aspect of the experience has been largely lost, as it always tends to be when original discriminations of the beyond and the personally initiated response thereto become stereotyped in a tradition and incorporated in an institution.

---

[1] *Op. cit.*, pp. 282-3.　　[2] *Op. cit.*, p. 293.　　[3] *Op. cit.*, p. 295.

II : *Fasting.* Concerning fasting Radin says :

' There are two things to be remembered in connection with it— first, that it is a method of superinducing a religious feeling ; and secondly, that this religious feeling in turn is bound up with the desire for preserving and perpetuating socio-economic life values. Among the Winnebago the desirability of the conditions superinduced by fasting lay not so much in the emotional pleasure it gave, although this is not to be underestimated, as in the belief which the shamans had developed, that such a state was essential for placing people in a position enabling them to overcome certain crises in life, which it was reasonable to believe might take place '.[1]

Dr. E. Westermarck, in discussing ' Restrictions in Diet ' made the observation :

' It is frequently adopted as a means of having supernatural converse or acquiring supernatural powers. He who fasts sees in dreams or visions things that no ordinary eye can see.'[2]

There is certainly abundant evidence among the Winnebago that fasting was an experimental method of getting into effective contact with the realm beyond, and the records of various fastings gathered by Radin afford excellent examples of the operation of fantasy thinking and experience in religion. The story concerning the origin of ' the Stench-Earth Medicine ' is extremely suggestive, and provides what is perhaps the key to the whole problem from one point of view. The story is that a certain man, suffering from consumption, got his friends to remove him into a separate lodge so that he might die alone. However, he was visited in his ' pitiable '[3] condition by birds and

---

[1] *Op. cit.*, p. 310.

[2] *The Origin and Development of the Moral Ideas*, ii, p. 292.

[3] To make oneself ' pitiable ' to the spirits seems to have been one of the conditions of blessing. Cf. Radin's footnote to p. 262 : ' According to general belief the spirits are supposed to have entered into a sort of " bargain " with the human beings by which they were to bestow their blessings upon them in exchange for tobacco, buckskins, and feathers. Of course, it must be understood that individuals must have the necessary requirements, such as a certain attitude of mind, fasting, etc., before their offering of tobacco has any meaning to the spirits.' In the account of

animals of various kinds, who all gave him medicine, and gradually cured him. Amongst them came the hitcara, who added a number of blessings, and said :

> ' Human ! you have dreamed, not only for yourself, but for all your descendants.'[1]

This passage is reminiscent of another, far better known :

> ' Your sons and your daughters shall prophesy, your old men shall dream dreams, and your young men shall see visions '.[2]

Truly, if it had not been for the ' dreaming ' of mankind, with all its transformations and interpretations of the world of sense perception, there would have been no religion, philosophy, or science.

But Radin is right in saying that it was not primarily for the purpose of the pleasure of seeing visions and dreaming dreams that the Winnebago took to fasting. It has already been shewn that there was a much more practical interest involved—that of becoming ' holy ' in the sense of successful, of securing blessings from the spirits by becoming ' pitiable '. Now fasting was the golden road to this kind of holiness. Radin gives the following significant extract from the Winnebago system of instruction :

> ' My son, when you grow up, you should try to be of some benefit to your fellowmen. There is only one way in which this can be done, and that is to fast. . . . If you thirst to death, the spirits who are in control of wars will bless you. . . . But, my son, if you do not fast repeatedly it will be all in vain that you inflict

' How Wegi'ceka tried to see Earthmaker,' on p. 291, we are told : ' Wegi'ceka made himself extremely " pitiable " and wept. . . . " Perhaps I will be able to see Earthmaker if I weep," he thought to himself.' And quite explicitly on p. 166, footnote, Radin comments on the phrase : ' See to it that they pity you,' thus : ' This is the regular expression used for blessing. The idea seems to be that through fasting and crying you are to put yourself in a " pitiable " condition and that then the spirits, seeing your state, will pity you and grant what you have asked.'

[1] Radin, *op. cit.*, p. 261.
[2] Joel, ch. ii, v. 28.

sufferings upon yourself. Blessings are not obtained except by making the proper offerings to the spirits and by putting yourself, time and again, in the proper mental condition. . . . If you do not obtain a spirit to strengthen you, you will amount to nothing in the estimation of your fellowmen, and they will show you little respect. . . . My son, as you travel along life's path, you will find many narrow passages (i.e., crises), and you can never tell when you will come to them. Try to anticipate them, so that you will be endowed with sufficient strength (by obtaining powers from the spirits) to pass safely through these narrow passages '.[1]

There is no doubt about the manner in which fasting affected the Winnebago ; it induced a condition of intense fantasy thinking. If fantasies of the auspicious appearance of spirits, or of satisfactory promises from them, resulted, the faster had gained his blessing and could no doubt face the future, and especially life's ' narrow passages ' with confidence. Radin says, in connection with the belief in spirits :

' To the average Winnebago the world is peopled by an indefinite number of spirits who manifest their existence in many ways, being either visible, audible, felt emotionally, or manifesting themselves by some sign or result. From a certain point of view all the spirits demonstrate their existence by the result, by the fact that the blessings they bestow upon man enable him to be successful, and this holds just as much for the spirit who manifests himself in the most intangible, emotional manner as for that one who is visible to man '.[2]

The emphasis upon the reality of that which can be an object of the mind is further illustrated in connection with the importance attributed to mental concentration :

' To the religiously inclined Winnebago the efficacy of a blessing of a ceremony, etc., depended upon what they called " concentraing one's mind " upon the spirits, upon the details of the ritual, or upon the precise purpose to be accomplished. All other thoughts were to be rigidly excluded, they believed. This was

[1] *Op. cit.*, pp. 277-8. The full account of the System of Instruction is to be found beginning at page 166.
[2] *Op. cit.*, p. 284.

the insistent admonition of the Winnebago elders to the youth
who was fasting. He was to center his mind completely on
the spirits, for his blessing would be in direct proportion to the
power of contentration he was capable of. The Winnebago
believed that the relation between man and the spirits was established by this concentration and that no manner of care in
ritualistic detail could take its place. Very frequently failure
on a warpath or lack of efficacy of a ritual was attributed to the
fact that the Indian or Indians had been lacking in the intensity
of their " concentration " '.[1]

This means that what, according to the theory advocated,
was originally an addition to or projection upon situations
characterized by ' beyond ' features—namely fantastic and
imaginative elements—tend to become detached from
specific things and situations, and to become generalized.
In that process, indeed, we may see the psychological
aspect of the birth of the gods. Accordingly, it becomes
natural for the religious man no longer merely to make the
religious response to specific situations and on occasions
when he is actually confronted with the impingement of
the ' beyond ', but to make opportunities of securing the
aid of the ' something more ' which has come to be recognized as more or less continuously present in all experience,
and has become at least partially accessible through special
modes of approach. That one of the most universal and
enduring of these modes should be that of fasting and
asceticism in general indicates how fundamental in religion
is the element of imaginative quickening which makes it
possible to ' see the invisible ' and to ' hear the inaudible'.

It now remains to shew that this interpretation of the
means by which fasting secured such great blessings is
supported by definite evidence. Radin provides it in
abundance in his collection of fasting experiences.

[1] *Op. cit.*, pp. 310-11.

(1) It is very clearly brought out in the example of *Personal Religious Experiences*, entitled ' How Wegi'ceka tried to see Earthmaker ' (already referred to above). The father urged his son to fast, and told him that Earthmaker must be ' in charge ' of much more power than other spirits, since it was he who had put them all in charge of something :

> ' Thus the old man reasoned and his son thought the same. So he tried to " dream " of Earthmaker. " I wonder what sort of blessings Earthmaker bestows on people ", he thought to himself.
> ' None of the spirits blessed Wegi'ceka during his fastings. He was always thinking of Earthmaker and asking him to bless him. Wegi'ceka made himself extremely " pitiable " and wept '.[1]

For a long time his efforts were unavailing. He married, and his wife assisted him in his efforts to ' dream ' of Earthmaker, even to the point of offering their first-born child as a sacrifice. Then visions began to come—but they were false ones (illusions, and not hallucinatory visions). Three times he saw, in different guise, what he thought was Earthmaker, and heard him speak ; but each time it turned out to have been a bird.

> ' Then for the last time he tried to " dream " of Earthmaker . . . He fasted, and soon Earthmaker, far above, heard his voice and said, " Wegi'ceka, you are weeping bitterly. For your sake I will come to the earth ". Then Earthmaker told Wegi'ceka that when he (Wegi'ceka) looked at him he would see a ray of light extending from above far down to his camp. That far it would reach. " Only thus, Wegi'ceka, can you see me. What you ask of me (to see me face to face) I cannot grant you. But, nevertheless, you may tell (your fellowmen) that you saw me ". Thus he spoke to him. He did not bless him with war powers. Only with life did he bless him '.[2]

(2) The account of J's fasting. He was told many things after much fasting.

[1] *Op. cit.*, p. 291. [2] *Op. cit.*, pp. 292-3.

' And this they told me about the ghost village—that when
I go there I will be able to steal a costly shawl from the spirits
and be able to escape with it ; that then all the inhabitants of
the ghost village would chase me, but that they would not be able
to overtake me and would be compelled to turn back as soon
I reached to earth . . .

' Now, all that I have spoken of, I dreamed. I really dreamed
that I was stealing a costly shawl and that I would have plenty
of them all the time. I dreamed that I would obtain ten or even
more shawls in one year and that I would not have to pay anything
for them. What the spirits meant by shawls was supplies. However, all this took place before I ate the peyote. Since then I
know that these things were not true, and that what I must
depend upon is not supernatural power, but myself, and my own
endeavours. Supernatural powers do not come from anywhere.
They do not exist at all. The blessings I had received were not
holy and I am not holy. This I know now. The whole thing is
untrue. Therefore I stopped using these supernatural powers
some time ago '.[1]

(3) How a bear blessed a man.

' Once a band of Winnebago used to give a feast to the bears.
A bear had blessed one of their number with life and victory on
the warpath.

' It was a spirit-bear that had blessed him . . .'[2]

It spoke to him and promised him certain conditional
advantages, with the details of which we are not here
concerned. The important point is the description of the
experience :

' This is what the man " dreamed ". He believed it and was
happy '.

(4) How the daughter of Mank'erexka refused a blessing
from Disease-giver.

The daughter of Mank'erexka fasted and received the
blessing of a deer. When, however, the deer came it was
killed by others, and the girl refused to eat,

---

[1] *Op. cit.*, p. 294.   [2] *Op. cit.*, p. 301.

' Then she rubbed some charcoal on her face and went to the place of fasting and said, " What you (the spirits) gave me others have taken away and eaten ". Early in the morning she looked around toward the water. She was very weak, for she had not eaten for a long time. Nine days she fasted. She was saying to herself, " As soon as I see a deer I will tell the others and call my father ". In the morning she went out in search of the deer. She was so weak that she could hardly crawl along. But she managed to reach the edge of the waters and, as she looked across, she saw a deer coming. So she immediately went to her father and told him. He got up immediately and, taking a spear, jumped into a boat, pursued, and speared it. Then the girl said, " Now I will eat ". So they called her uncles, Wolf and Elk. When they came she put tobacco in their hands and said, " My uncles, I have offered tobacco to the different spirits and asked them to bless me. Now I am about to eat and I would like to have you put some food into your mouths ". " My niece, it is good. You have indeed made yourself ' pitiable '. You have thirsted yourself to death and I, too, pity you. If any spirit has blessed you he has done so with good reason. I, too, once thirsted myself to death and the spirits blessed me with life. With this life, my niece, I also bless you. I will gladly partake of your feast, " Thus spoke Wolf. Then Elk said, " My niece, I, too, was told to fast ; and in my fast the spirits blessed me with the power of having complete control over all my actions. This dream (i.e., the blessing I obtained) I now give to you. With these blessings you will be able to live as you desire. I will now gladly partake of your food ".

' When they were through eating, she also ate, and then they all went home. After a while her father said to her, " My daughter, I am going to ask you a question. It is said that those who have been blessed might tell their dreams if they were asked ". " All right ", said the daughter, " I will tell you. Eight days I fasted and then the spirits blessed me. They told me that if at the end of four days I should place offerings south of the place known as the Big Eddy, and situated down the stream, the powers with which I had been blessed would be shown to me. The one who blessed me was the chief of the Wak^{e}ai^{n}tcu^n the spirits who live in the earth. He said that Earthmaker had created him and given him great power ; that he had placed him in charge of ' life '. In four days he told me, ' I will appear to you. The day on which I appear to you will be a perfect day. Whatever you wish to make for yourself, you may do. You will never be in want of anything, for you can make implements for yourself out of my body. With these I bless you, for you have made yourself suffer very much, and my heart has been rent with pity for you. I will bless you, therefore, with life, and this you may transmit to your descendants '. All this, father, the spirit said

to me ". " My daughter, it is not good. These spirits are trying
to deceive you. Do not accèpt it. They will never bestow upon
you what they have promised ". " All right, father, but let me
at least give them the offerings of deerskin, red feathers, and
tobacco. I will not accept these blessings, for you forbid it ".
‘ Then after four days she took her offerings to the place where
she was to meet the spirit and told him that her father had forbidden her to accept the blessing. " ' You are not a good spirit ',
he said ". " He is right, for one side of my body is not good
but the other is ", answered the spirit. " This is the way in
which Earthmaker created me ". Thus the wak^{e}ai^{n}tcu^n; spoke.
Then the woman looked toward the lake and she saw a tree standing
in the water. The spirit climbed upon this tree and wrapped
himself around it. Then he took a tooth and shot the tree and
knocked it down. " This is what you would have been able to
do ", said the spirit. " The people would have respected you
very much. You would have been able to cure weak or nervous
people. But you did not listen to what I told you. You refused
it " '.[1]

This story has been quoted in full because it displays, in
addition to the function of the ' dream ' in attaining holiness and blessing, the ' transference ' of blessings, and also
the safeguards surrounding the validity of these dream
experiences—a point which will receive attention shortly.
Concerning the transference of the uncles' blessings, Radin
says in a footnote :

‘ The transference of certain blessings is very common, but, to
my knowledge, it is rarely done in this manner. As a rule if a
person was unable to obtain blessings, he sought to offset this
handicap in life by purchasing supernatural powers from some of
his more successful fellowmen. However, these powers seem to
be connected almost exclusively with medicines. That blessings
such as those bestowed upon individuals during their fast, such
as long life, invincibility, hunting powers, etc., were transferred,
does not seem probable, although it is, of course, possible. The
writer was told of a number of cases where this seemed to have
been the case, but on closer study it was conclusively shown that
no real transference had taken place, but that in those instances
where a person had said, " I transfer this and that dream to you ",
the transference had no validity unless the individual to whom
the dream had been bequeathed actually fasted and obtained
the same dream. An individual would in such a case always be

[1] *Op cit.*, pp. 302-4.

careful to select as his " dream-heir " one who would in all likelihood obtain the same dream. It is only in this sense that one
might actually speak of a transference. In those instances where
a man is blessed with supernatural powers that are to extend
to all his posterity this is what is really meant, namely, an infinite
repetition of the same blessing, one that has, however, become so
certain within definite families that it might be considered automatic '.[1]

Thus fasting is the recognized means of securing personal
contact with the spirits by means of dreaming—that is,
fantasy thinking of hallucinatory vividness. Its survival
as a successful method of approach to the ' beyond ' is
evidence of three things. (i) It points to the fundamental
character of fantasy in the religious response. (ii) It
indicates that there must be some recognized relationship
between the fantasy and the established order of reality—
it must not merely provide an ' escape from reality '. We
have just seen that in the story of Mank'erexka's daughter,
the girl is forbidden to take her dream seriously by her
father, on the ground that the ' spirits are trying to deceive '
and that ' they will never bestow ' what they have promised. Her fantasies, in short, had taken her so far beyond
the range of legitimate expectation as to be declared unreal
even by a believer in the blessings of the spirits. The
principle is again illustrated in the story of Y's fasting,
which may usefully be quoted : at one time, we are told,
the Winnebago had no war-bundle while other tribes had,
so

' K'erex^{e}u^{n}'sak'a started to fast for one. He fasted from
early autumn until summer and he received a blessing. Then
he went to his father and told him, " Father, you told me to fast.
Let us now go and see with what I have been blessed ". So the
old man accompanied his son. When the old man got there he
found a snake dried and dressed up and standing in an upright
position. The snake had long hairs on its back, scattered here and

---

[1] *Op. cit.*, p. 303 (f-n).

there. The father on seeing it said, " My son, this is really too great. If you accept this and carry it with you on the warpath, you will not leave any human beings alive (i.e., you will always want to go on the warpath) ". The son therefore refused it, and went out to fast again. Then the spirits blessed him again and again he went to his father and asked to accompany him to the wilderness and see what blessings he had obtained. When they came to the wilderness they found two wild cats (already stuffed) standing there and facing in opposite directions. Then the old man told his son again not to accept this blessing because it would be too powerful, but the young man said, " This is the last blessing that I am going to get ", and accepted it '.[1]

Radin makes the following comments in a footnote to this story :

' By " too powerful " the old man means that the feasts, offerings, etc., that would be necessary for so great a blessing would be quite beyond the means or ability of the young man. It is to be remembered that the bestowal of a blessing does not in itself insure its efficacy, but that this can only be assured if the proper offerings and the proper emotional attitude accompany its subsequent use. Evidently the old man did not feel that the young fellow would be equal to the task. I have been told by many of the older Winnebagoes that when the old system was still intact the older people always made it a point to warn impetuous youths against taking upon themselves responsibilities that they might possibly not be able to fulfil, a very excellent device, it seems to me, for not multiplying the chance of failures and consequently the necessity of explaining them. However, one need not believe that this was the reason for their caution '.[2]

It does not seem to me to indicate ' caution ' in the sense Radin suggests at all, but rather a definite recognition that any ' dream ' that is quite out of touch with possibilities as recognized in the order of reality accepted must be discountenanced. Religion, in a word, has to do with that which is ' beyond ', but it must deal with it in such a way as to relate it practically with life, if only through a suggestive reinforcement of self-confidence. To accept a dream of benefits which contradict the order of reality as recog-

[1] *Op. cit.*, pp. 299-300.   [2] *Op. cit.*, p. 300 (f-n).

nized is obviously to court failure ; hence the tendency to attribute such ' dreams ' to the deceitfulness of spirits or to bad spirits. (iii) It emphasizes the fact that there are inevitably situations to be faced which are of a ' beyond ' character—not to be dealt with by man's ordinary capacities, and that it is necessary to fortify oneself against these crises or ' narrow passages '—that is, to learn the way of religious response as a personal experience, or else, failing that, to buy such immunity as may be had from experts. Inability to discriminate the ' beyond ' situation and to overcome the experience of frustration resulting therefrom by successful dream interpretations incapacitates a man from being religious in the first-hand or primary sense— and he must do the best he can by other methods.

Fantasy supervening upon intensely affective experience of beyondness or ' utter-otherness ', which enables the worshipper or devotee to face his environment with confidence and hope, has obvious psychological value. We are not here concerned with the question of its objective reference. That there is something more in the universe than those familiar characteristics which can be directly responded to by native powers of reaction, and that this something is vaguely discriminated in what are primarily feeling experiences, seems beyond question. But equally obviously the psychologist can only judge the attempt to reduce this element to fantastic, imaginative, ideational or conceptual form from the point of view of psychological success, not of epistemological validity. But this does not imply that fantasy and dream elements are ' unreal ', as Durkheim supposes in the following passage :

' Nothing is worth nothing. The impressions produced in us by the physical world can, by definition, contain nothing that surpasses this world. Out of the visible, only the visible can be made ; out of that which is heard, we cannot make something not heard. Then to explain how the idea of sacredness has been able to take form under these conditions, the majority of the theorists have been obliged to admit that men have super-imposed upon reality, such as it is given by observation, an unreal world, constructed entirely out of the fantastic images which agitate his mind during a dream, or else out of the frequently monstrous aberrations produced by the mythological imagination under the bewitching but deceiving use of language. But it remained incomprehensible that humanity should have remained obstinate in these errors through the ages, for experience should have very quickly proven them false '.[1]

For we may note the following facts : (i) Impressions produced by the physical world can and do contain what surpasses the world ' such as it is given to observation ' at any point where they stimulate fantasy and imagination. Durkheim's formula, in fact, could only hold if perception were identical with ' pure sensation '. The world is not ' given ' but, at least in large measure, fabricated by ' observation '. (ii) Fantasy is not something that is borrowed from dreams. Dreams are one form of fantasy thinking, and fantasy is itself a mental response. Whether we accept the Freudian formulation or prefer that of Rivers, the dream is essentially the expression of thwarted tendencies. The most frequent stimulus to day-dreaming is the

---

[1] The *Elementary Forms of the Religious Life*, p. 225. In this instance Lévy-Bruhl may be effectively set against Durkheim. In *Primitive Mentality*, Geo. Allen and Unwin, 1923, p. 60, speaking of the manner in which the primitive represents to himself mystic force in what is presented to his senses, he says : ' Undoubtedly this kind of intuition does not make it possible to perceive the invisible or touch the intangible ; it cannot have the effect of giving sense-perception of what is outside the realm of sense. But it does give implicit faith in *the presence and agency* of powers which are invisible and inaccessible to the senses, and this certainly equals, if it does not surpass, that afforded by the senses themselves. To the pre-logical mind these elements of reality—much the most important in his eyes—are no less matters of fact than the others.' These elements of reality, it should be added, are not only matters of fact to ' pre-logical ' mentality, if such a stage can be said to exist, but also to logical mentality : it is only a difference determined by environmental factors and the extent of practical knowledge that separates the primitive savage from the civilized scientist or theologian.

thwarting of tendencies by the environment. It is entirely unpsychological to dismiss fantasy, whether in dream or day-dream, as mere agitation of mind which has no relation to reality. It plays a very important part in constituting reality as experienced. (iii) The ' errors ' under which man has laboured as a result of his fantasies are not explained by Durkheim's own purely sociological theory of religion. The facts of the matter are, (a) that the ' errors ' are corrected as knowledge advances, and (b) that the ' errors ' persist while they provide more adequate outlet to mental activity which would otherwise be thwarted, than alternative formulations. Many ' errors ' are—as Durkheim himself has to suppose for the purposes of his theory—pragmatic ' truths '.

III. The Spirits and Earthmaker. Concerning the Winnebago attitude to the Spirits in general Radin says :

' Those Indians who have never spent any time thinking upon the nature of spirits can not truly be said to have any concept of their nature, whether vague or definite. They simply repeat what they have heard from the more religiously inclined. An answer prompted by a moment's consideration, as is often the case when an ethnologist interrogates them, does not necessarily reflect the current view of the subject, nor, for that matter, even the same Indian's belief after he has given the matter some thought. Many Winnebago, with whom the author was fairly well acquainted, refused to answer certain questions offhand, and asked for time to reflect about them. It seems justified, when we are studying a subject like religion, to ask for information from those who have, in all probability, formulated the beliefs—the shamans. It is from them we must strive to learn whether the spirits are conceived of as anthropomorphic, theromorphic, dream-phantasms, or indefinite entities in general.

' In trying to discover this the author found, not only that he was asking a leading question, but that he was asking an unnecessary question. It was soon quite clear that the Winnebago did not base their test of the existence of a spirit on the presence or absence of corporeality ; in other words, upon such sense perceptions as sight and hearing. It is because we Europeans do insist that the presence or absence of corporeality is the test of reality or unreality that we have been led to make the classification into personal and impersonal. But the Winnebago apparently does not insist that existence depends upon sense perceptions alone. He claims that what is thought of, what is felt' and what is spoken, in fact, anything that is brought before his consciousness, is a sufficient indication of its existence and it is the question of the existence and reality of these spirits in which he is interested. The question of their corporeality is of comparative unimportance and most of the questions connected with the personal or impersonal nature of the spirits do not exist.

' It is clear that if comparatively little stress has been laid by the Winnebago on the personality of the spirits, it will be difficult to define them precisely except by their names, by their attributes, and by the nature of the blessings which they bestow on man. What seems to stand out most prominently in the attitude of the Winnebago toward their spirits is the intense belief in the reality of their existence, which is due first to what might be called the " emotional authority " for their existence, and secondly, to the fact that the life values of man are intensely real and the spirits are theoretically in control of these life values.

' To the average Winnebago the world is peopled by an indefinite number of spirits who manifest their existence in many ways, being either visible, audible, felt emotionally, or manifesting themselves by some sign or result. From a certain point of view all the spirits demonstrate their existence by the result, by the fact that the blessings they bestow upon man enable him to be successful, and this holds just as much for the spirit who manifests himself in the most intangible, emotional manner as for that one who is visible to man '.[1]

Probably what Radin means when he speaks of the absence of stress on the ' personality ' of the spirits is what we ordinarily mean by individuality. There may be little to distinguish the character of one spirit from another, but that does not mean that they are not endowed with the value of personality. On the contrary it is quite clear that with the Winnebago the spirits are personifications connected with life values, arrived at through the projection of fantasy and image. Radin himself is very emphatic that among the Winnebago there is no general

[1] 37th. An. Rep. Am. Bur. Ethn., pp. 283-4.

idea of the supernatural as a force or energy of an impersonal character :

> ' The Winnebago have no such belief in a " magic power " as Mr. J. N. B. Hewitt and Mr. W. Jones would have us believe exists among the Iroquois and Fox . . . we have given our reasons for believing that these ethnologists were mistaken in their interpretation '.[1]

If the spirits, then, are not departments of *orenda, manito, wakan*, or *mana*, and yet are given names, have offerings and fasts and prayers made to them, it is difficult to deny them personality, though there may be no clear-cut theory of the personal nature of the spirits.

Radin attributes the ' intense belief in the reality ' of the spirits to (i) ' the " emotional authority " for their existence ', and (ii) ' the fact that the life values of man are intensely real and the spirits are theoretically in control of these life values '. To these should be added the factor, already referred to, that, according to Radin, for the Winnebago ' anything that is brought before his consciousness is a sufficient indication of its existence '— though in regard to the precise significance of this statement it would be desirable to have fuller information. I suspect that the fact is that it is whatever is brought before consciousness with what Hume described as ' the force and

---

[1] *Op. cit.*, p. 283. It may be noted that Durkheim assumes the validity of the idea of a pre-eminent impersonal power among ' primitives.' Thus on p. 192-3 (*Elem. Forms*) ' . . . there is (among the Sioux) the pre-eminent power to which all the others have the relation of derived forms, and which is called *wakan* . . . the *wakan* is in no way a personal being,' etc. ' Among the Iroquois . . . this same idea is found again ; the word *orenda* which expresses it being the exact equivalent of the *wakan* of the Sioux.' Also James H. Leuba, *A Psychological Study of Religion*, 1912, pp. 70-84. Leuba quotes Irving King for confirmation of the view that ' the terms *Manitou* (Algonquin) *Wakonda* (Sioux), *Orenda* (Iroquois), *Mana* (Melanesian), designate a non-personal Power or Potency considered to be at the basis of all natural phenomena. The same notion is found among the Australians.' Reference may also be made to R. R. Marett, *The Threshold of Religion*, where he treats *mana* as ' that positive emotional value which is the raw material of religion, and only needs to be moralized . . . to become its essence.'

vivacity' of an 'original sentiment'[1] that is taken as being 'real', precisely because there is nothing to distinguish it from a perception so far as the experient is concerned. It is difficult to believe that the Winnebago are incapable of having mental imagery which they recognize as such, and which they would not treat as self-evident proof of the existence of the imaged thing. The earnestness with which fasting is practised in order that definite dreams and visions may result (which have the 'force and vivacity' of an 'original sentiment') shews that it is what comes into consciousness with the usual signs of objectivity that is accepted as real. Any Winnebago, presumably, could casually imagine one of the spirits blessing him; but to gain the blessing, in fact, concentration resulting in imagination of hallucinatory vividness is necessary.[2]

Thus the psychological mechanism involved in the birth and development of the Winnebago spirits is undoubtedly fantasy initiated by frustration experience. The growth of the power of recognizing 'life values' is accompanied by an increasing discrimination of elements in connection with these values which do not directly or immediately yield themselves to ordinary treatment and manipulation. The tendencies in their normal functioning do not carry man to the fulfilment of his needs, enlarged as these constantly are by his fuller discriminations. Thwarted by his environment he (i) experiences affect and (ii) projects fantasies upon the situation. He must account for the mystery of the elusiveness of the objects of his desire and of his experience—account for them, that is, so far as to bring

---

[1] *An Enquiry Concerning Human Understanding*, Section ii.
[2] See above, p. 71-2—quotation from Radin on Concentration. Cf. also the whole discussion of fasting and its relation to dream fantasies above, pp. 69-78.

himself into experimental relations with them—or else he must repress his consciousness of and interest in everything that falls beyond his reach, which is to sacrifice that which is distinctively human. To refer particular departments of nature, or special life values, to spirits or gods, is a development of the more vague and emotional response to the mysterious and ' beyond ' and uncanny which cannot be put into intellectual terms without distortion, but which can still be experienced by modern man, in spite of sophistication. The eerie feeling that most of us experience in walking through a lonely and isolated cemetery at midnight or amid the mists of early dawn, the chilling sense of the uncanny that lingers after hearing ' ghost stories ' well told by an imaginative raconteur, the inexplicable and unutterable feelings that sometimes haunt us in vast untenanted spaces or in dense forests, all display one aspect of the primitive religious response. To refer the emotional disturbance induced by a pressure upon, or invasion of, consciousness of the mysterious, the inaccessible, the uncanny, to a ' presence ', a spirit, or magic force, is simply a matter of conceptualizing the experience. The spirit is the verbal or ideational symbol for the experience of conscious contact with something that is beyond the range of the normal tendencies. The primordial fact is the mystery, which breaks in in various ways upon consciousness as it develops and becomes receptive to reality in ways which are not associated with hereditary or acquired tendencies to action. In the evolution of religion we pass from the first vague and chaotic experience of the mysterious in particular instances to fantastic interpretation (or distortion), through more controlled imaginative interpretation to the phase of philosophical and theological reflection. The earliest type of response to sporadic impingements of the mysterious upon consciousness is probably something which defies our attempts at exact specification—it belongs to a ' pre-magical ' as well as a ' pre-animistic ' phase.[1] If we could get the introspective account of a cat's or dog's experience at a time when one of these animals suddenly displays in a quiet room all the signs of awareness of an invisible somewhat which is uncanny, we might learn much concerning the nature of the primitive religious response. When a magician or medicine-man arises as the practitioner of hurt and healing through the manipulation of what we should call ' occult ' forces, the religious response has undergone considerable development through interpretation. This applies still more to the phase of animism and polytheism. The religion of the Winnebago, as described by Radin, presents us with the interesting and instructive ' moment ' in religious evolution when the primary experience of the mysterious has been classified and personified, and is well on the way to being rationalized in respectable monistic terms. Particular domains of the mysterious, as it affects various life values, are referred to spirits ; but all these spirits are in the stage of being subordinated to Earthmaker, who is the ultimate creator of everything. To the spirits he has delegated control over various things which he has created. Given the pressure of the same environmental factors, it is probable that just as the Hebrews passed from polytheism to henotheism and thence to monotheism, so would the Winnebago. When reflection reaches the conclusion that all mysterious manifestations are the expressions of one and

---

[1] R. R. Marett, *op. cit.*, discusses ' pre-animistic religion ' in the first chapter.

the same force, and not separate entities, the way is open for monotheism.

IV. *Contact with the white man.* The story of the Decora family is of value and interest in shewing the emergence of new religious tendencies. The reaction of the Winnebago to the French was clearly of the submissive or receptive type. The new values of various kinds (if only in purely material arts) to which they were introduced by the French were appreciated and desired. Accordingly the marriage of the Frenchman Decora with the daughter of the chief seems to have been welcomed, and peculiar respect and regard paid to the two children of the marriage, for they might be expected to guide and help the community to reap the advantages of the new situation involved in the presence of the various influences of white civilization. Naturally, then, ' the Indians made them fast ', for in this way they would secure the blessings which would make them invaluable to the group. The casting out of the elder son by the uncle because he tried ' to eat some corn ' was disapproved by the group, and attributed to personal fear on the part of the uncle, shewing that already there was a new orientation in process. The boy, who was the son of the powerful Frenchman, was not to be judged by ordinary standards, applicable to the Winnebago. Thus on his return he was endowed with great prestige, which enabled him, apparently without opposition, to introduce the drum, with which Earthmaker had blessed him, and to become a leader. And the implication is that his leadership was one of no mere secular character, but partook of the nature of religious and prophetic authority.

' He was called to take the foremost part in everything. . . . Only they (the Decora family) could accomplish anything among the whites . . . the object that he said was sacred (the drum) is indeed sacred. It is powerful to the present day '.

It matters relatively little whether the incidents are actually historical in detail or not—whether Decora's son actually introduced the drum, or whether this account of so important a part of the religious regalia of the Winnebago was really an origin myth ; in either case it displays the attitude of the Winnebago as one of receptivity to the new influences brought by the coming of the white man, and a receptivity which has the characteristics of a religious attitude, in as much as new methods of approach to the ' beyond ' elements as represented, e.g. by Earthmaker, are derived from this person of French extraction.

Radin goes on to comment upon the fact that prophecy seems to have been one of the direct outcomes of the contact with the whites :

> ' One of the interesting developments resulting from the Indian contact with the whites has been the appearance of prophets. In almost all cases these prophets were concerned with attempts to so adapt the life of their fellow-Indians to the new conditions that they would be better able to cope with the invaders who were sweeping all before them. Whether prophets sprang up only in response to the peculiar conditions resulting from the presence of the whites it is impossible to say, but there seems no reason to believe that such had always been the case. It is quite possible that conditions similar to those developing from the occupancy of America by Europeans had occurred in pre-Columbian times when one tribe was hard pressed by another '.[1]

Prophecy in general is to be regarded as a new outburst of religious activity : its burden may be a recall to the ancient ways, or a summons to new ways of life, but in either case it is a protest against the inadequacy of present and existing adaptation to environment. Moreover, it involves the recognition that no secular methods of adaptation will suffice in face of the situation which is developing. In

[1] 37th. An. Rep. Am. Bur. Ethn., p. 69.

other words, existing organization of the response-tendencies gives way, proves inadequate, before a situation which is characterized by elements of the unfamiliar and mysterious. The response to such a situation is that process of interpretation which has already been described at some length. The prophet is the person whose dreams, visions and imaginings in relation to the strange situation are of a nature to help bring it within the scope of some kind of effort at practical adaptation. The threat of uncontrollable forces, whether of disease, famine, invasion or natural convulsion, may lead to the imaginative interpretation of an outraged deity whose commandments have been disobeyed, and who thus exerts his mysterious power to recall—or at any rate warn—his disobedient people. Or these threats may be interpreted as signs that some new system of ceremony or belief is required by the deity if he is not to cast off his people utterly. The whole development of Hebrew prophecy is an illustration of this process, with the emphasis upon the restoration of a supposedly purer worship which existed in the past. Adaptation to the mysterious reality and power of Yahweh (which would bring success and well-being to the Hebrew world) was a *return* in theory to the pristine purity and excellence of early days. In fact, of course, the demands of the Hebrew prophets were largely new interpretations of religious and ceremonial duty, for the golden age of the past was as much a dream as the resplendent visions of the future were.

In the case of the Shawnee prophet, of whom Radin gives an account[1], there is a recognition of both requirements.

' " Let the people give up the customs they are now observing and I will give them new ones ". This is what he said '.

[1] *Op. cit.*, pp. 69-74.

But the result was that

> ' some of the Winnebago did this and threw away their war bundles. But he had meant their bad customs. Some also threw away their good medicines '.

So a deputation of the Winnebago waited on the prophet to learn what really was necessary :

> ' Younger brothers, we are not doing the right thing, and that is why we are not getting along very well in life '.

he told them. But what ' not doing the right thing ' involved was not merely observing old customs which they ought to give up for new ones, for the prophet also said :

> ' that he had been sent by the Creator because the Indians were wandering away from their old customs. For that reason the Creator had sent him to tell them of it '.

As a general principle it may be said to be expedient to recommend new customs as if they were old ones which have been neglected, for in all groups with an established tradition the conservative and resistive tendencies are stronger than the creative. It is for this reason that most of the sects of Christianity claim for their special witness or practices that they are ' primitive and apolostolical ' (in John Wesley's phrase),[1] and that they represent a return to New Testament teaching and intention.

It is of interest and importance to note in connection with the Shawnee prophet that even in the brief account given of his career there are abundant signs of mental instability.[2] This, indeed, it may confidently be asserted,

---

[1] ' I dare not presume to impose my mode of worship on any other. I believe it is truly primitive and apostolical. But my belief is no rule for another.' From a Sermon, quoted in *A Book of Devotional Readings*, edited by J. M. Connell, 1913, p. 191.

[2] See Radin's account on pp. 70-1. The prophet forgets his mission ' for the devil misrepresented things to him and he believed him '; he has numerous communications with the devil ; is subject to fits of anger, attaining on occasions murderous intensity ; frequently gets drunk ; is unkind to women, who nevertheless go with him through the attraction of fear ; is recalled to his mission by hearing the voice of the Creator, and by seeing numerous visions, not specially induced by such recognized methods as fasting, but arising spontaneously.

is one of the indispensable conditions of prophecy. The
mentally stable, or resistive person,[1] faced with a crisis,
can do no more than respond to it along the lines of his
established tendencies. He simply ' carries on ' in the old-
established ways, and either lives through the crisis by
ignoring whatever in it does not yield to customary modes
of behaviour, or succumbs precisely because he lacks the
mental plasticity to effect a new orientation and initiate
fresh modes of response. The prophet, on the other hand,
discerns in crisis a situation with ' beyond ' elements which
must be met by changed methods of response, and his
discernment is made possible by the sensitiveness to
experience which easily becomes in unfavourable conditions
instability ; in other words, by the absence of fixity in his
mental mechanisms. It is for this reason that insanity
has so frequently been regarded among various peoples as
possession by the deity : a person capable of such unusual
behaviour, and subject to such novel impulsions, is obviously in closer contact with the uncanny powers of mystery.
Speaking of the popular exclamation (1 Samuel x. v. 11),
' Is Saul also among the prophets ? ' A. B. Davidson says
that it

> ' has been taken as an expression of wonder that a solid yeoman
> like Saul should join himself to a company of ranting enthusiasts.
> This view is wholly improbable. It was not in this way that
> religious exaltation was looked upon in the East. It was just

[1] W. Trotter, in *Instincts of the Herd in Peace and in War*, has made the
suggestive classification of types into the ' stable-minded, conservative
and resistive ' on the one hand, and the ' mentally unstable ' on the other.
These latter have a greater sensibility to the suggestions of experience
(as distinguished from suggestions issuing from the herd). This type, he
points out, are very adaptable but lacking in the solid virtues of the re-
sistives. ' The pressing problem which . . . faces man in the immediate
future is how to readjust the mental environment in such a way that
sensitiveness may develop and confer on man the enormous advantages
which it holds for him, without being transformed from a blessing into
the curse and menace of instability.' (p. 64)

the visible excitation that suggested to the onlooker that the enthusiast was possessed by the deity. Even the insane, just because he had no mastery over his mind, which seemed moved by another, was held inspired '.[1]

We may be sure that the experience of contact with the whites did not of itself call into existence a mental plasticity or instability which was not there before. Probably among all peoples at all times there are certain individuals in whom there are ' difference tendencies ' strongly marked who display behaviour which is unusual and unconventional according to prevailing standards, and in whom there is a greater measure of plasticity or adaptability. But the innovator or prophet is not welcomed or regarded in a time of prosperity and comfort when the established contacts with reality are proving adequate for group maintenance. Thus while a period of crisis, a new and unfamiliar situation, does not call into existence a new psychological type, it does provide the conditions under which the more sensitive and potentially unstable type may come into social prominence and even favour—because they alone have any fresh guidance to offer in the face of conditions which baffle the stable and resistive type. It may well happen that the community at large may remain insensitive to the new situation in spite of the warnings of the few, and prefer to muddle through on the lines of established behaviour patterns.[2] The prophet then experiences misunderstanding, persecution, rejection and often death. But in fact

[1] Hastings' *Dictionary of the Bible*, 5th Impression, 1905, vol. iv, Art. *Prophecy and Prophets*, pp. 109-10.

[2] Principal John W. Graham, in an Article on George Fox in *The Hibbert Journal*, vol. xxii, no. 4, speaking of the conditions when Fox was preaching makes the observation : ' Should a great religious genius arise, the fields were indeed white unto harvest. Much would depend on the man appearing. It has been our world calamity that in the War of 1914, and the period of disasters it has left, no great man, no man great enough for the task, has been in effective power for long in any State.'

he is simply doing afresh what the old forms of religion had come into existence to do, namely, to effect a *modus vivendi* with the world conditions as they are enlarged and amplified to an expanding capacity of discrimination. It would seem, therefore, that the conditions for the fresh outburst of religion are similar to those which we must suppose to be implicit from the earliest dawn of religion : an appreciable experience of perplexity in the presence of baffling features in the environment, and the capacity on the part of some individual or individuals in the group to suggest a new mode of approach to the situation by reducing it through fantastic, imaginative, philosophical or theological interpretation to accessibility.

IV

THE PEYOTE CULT AMONG THE WINNEBAGO

THERE are two quite distinct questions in connection with the introduction of the Peyote Cult among the Winnebago, with the second of which alone I am directly concerned : (1) the psychological factors involved in the process of borrowing new elements of culture, and (2) the psychological factors involved in giving the cult a definitely religious character. From the point of view of the psychology of borrowing the fact that in this instance it is an element of religious culture which is borrowed is of secondary importance.[1] In his *Sketch of the Peyote Cult of the Winnebago*,[2] Dr. Radin is primarily concerned with the study of borrowing, not of religion, and accordingly there is more material illustrative of the psychology of borrowing than of the psychology of religion in these pages. Fortunately Dr. Radin has included a more general account of the Cult in his exhaustive monograph on the Winnebago Tribe, and it is from this source that the present chapter derives most of its material, supplemented occasionally by references to features which are peculiar to the *Sketch of the Peyote Cult*. The problem of this chapter may thus be stated :

[1] F. C. Bartlett, *Psychology and Primitive Culture*, p. 176, says : 'What are the kinds of detail which have most frequently been introduced into new settings in this way ? Articles of food and of dress, weapons of warfare, stories and myths, practices connected with material arts, ceremonial observances, religious beliefs, details of play.'

[2] *Journal of Religious Psychology*, vol. 7, Jan. 1914, no. 1, pp. 1-22.

What gives the Peyote Cult its religious character, and what is involved in the general Winnebago response to the new religion which differentiates it from a response to the introduction of a new element of art or other feature which might be borrowed ?

Mr. F. C. Bartlett in his use of Radin's material for a study in the psychology of borrowing, makes the following important statement :

> ' As to whether there are sufficient reasons for assuming a distinct religious instinct or not, we need not now inquire. But that there is a " religious interest, or bent ", original so far as the individual is concerned, stimulated by early training, but not wholly derived from this, and taking specific forms of development in different instances, seems to me indisputable. Rave, and I think also Hensley, show distinct evidence of the possession of such interest '.[1]

[1] *Psychology and Primitive Culture*, p. 175. A good instance of the operation of what looks like such an ' individual difference tendency ' or definitely religious ' interest or bent ' is afforded by St. Teresa (*The Life of St. Teresa*, written by herself, translated by Rev. John Dalton, 1851). She records that at a tender age she and her brother ' joined together in reading the Lives of the Saints. When I saw the martyrdoms through which many had passed, for the love of God, I thought they had purchased very cheaply, the sight and enjoyment of God ; and I myself felt a great desire to die in this manner ; *not*, however, through the love which I thought I had for him, but rather that I might, by so short a way, enjoy the possession of those immense goods which I had read were to be found in heaven. I, therefore, and my brother considered together, what means there were within our reach, for attaining this object. We agreed to go into the country of the Moors, and to beg our way for the love of God, so that we might be put to death there.' Being unable, owing to parental solicitude, to carry out this scheme, Teresa and her brother tried to become hermits in the garden. She also gave alms, tried to be much alone for devotions especially the rosary, and, ' I took great delight, when playing with other children, in making monasteries, as if we had been nuns ; and it seemed as if I desired to be one, though not so earnestly as I did those things of which I have spoken.' This seems to be a clear instance in which a certain peculiar direction of interest early made itself manifest. The youthful Teresa appears to have started life with an unusually marked capacity, or aptitude, for the vocation of a ' religious ' —an aptitude which in those days and in that environment naturally found expression in the life of a nun, but which might in these days, under appropriate environmental conditions, find expression in some form of religious, artistic, social or philanthropic activity. The point is that there definitely seems to be an impetus ' original so far as the individual is concerned,' as Bartlett says, which we must regard as a fundamental element in the personality of Teresa. This original impetus was ' stimulated by early training,' and directed by the pressure of social suggestion and the total environment, into the specific form of the monastic life.

With this important suggestion in mind I shall approach the problem of this chapter with an investigation into the personal experience of John Rave, who introduced the Cult among the Winnebago, in the light of such information as is available concerning the psychological make-up of his personality. It may then be possible to form some estimate of the nature of the original interest and its relation to other elements combining with this interest to give the Peyote Cult its religious character. I have already insisted that there is no justification for appealing to a ' religious instinct ', and the whole argument as already developed has aimed at shewing that religion derives its psychological character and peculiarity from the very fact that it transcends instinct endowment.

The main features of John Rave's life, so far as they enter into the Peyote conversion experience, are as follows :

' He was a member of the Bear clan, and had participated actively in all the prominent ceremonies, with the exception of the Medicine dance. He was thus thoroughly acquainted with the ritualistic and organization units '.[1]

He was reputed to have been

' . . . a bad man. He roamed from place to place. He has participated in all the ceremonies of the Winnebago, the medicine dance alone excepted. He had been married many times. Up to 1901 he was a heavy drinker. In that year he went to Oklahoma and while there ate the peyote. He then returned to the Winnebago and tried to introduce it among them, but none with the exception of a few relatives would have anything to do with it. This did not in any way discourage him, however, and he continued using the peyote, now and then getting a few converts '.[2]

There is a somewhat obscure reference to his wandering

---

[1] *Journal of Religious Psychology* (hereafter referred to as J.R.P.), vol. 7, no. 1, p. 20.
[2] 37th Annual Report of the American Bureau of Ethnology (hereafter A.R.A.B.E.), p. 394, from O.L.'s account.

propensities in the account of J.B., whom Radin describes as ' a very lukewarm follower ' :

'. . . when he reached middle age he began to travel around the world and learn different Indian languages. He used to travel inland a good deal. Once he joined a circus and crossed the ocean. . . . Shortly after this he travelled again and came to a band of Indians who were eating peyote. It was his custom to try everything when he went visiting. He did not realize what he was doing when he ate this medicine, but he did it anyhow '.[1]

In an autobiographical account of his conversion Rave himself concludes by saying :

' It is now 23 years since I first ate peyote, and I am still doing it (1912). Before that my heart was filled with murderous thoughts I wanted to kill my brother and my sister. It seemed to me that my heart would not feel good until I killed one of them. All my thoughts were fixed on the warpath. This is all I thought of. Now I know that it was because the evil spirit possessed me that I felt that way. I was suffering from a disease. I even desired to kill myself ; I did not care to live. That feeling, too, was caused by this evil spirit living within me. Then I ate this medicine and everything changed. The brother and sister I wanted to kill before I became attached to and I wanted them to live. The medicine had accomplished this '.[2]

We may now proceed to Rave's own account of the peyote and his religious experience :

' During 1893-94 I was in Oklahoma with peyote eaters. In the middle of the night we were to eat peyote. We ate it and I also did. It was the middle of the night when I got frightened, for a live thing seemed to have entered me. " Why did I do it ? " I thought to myself. I should not have done it, for right at the beginning I have harmed myself. Indeed, I should not have done it. I am sure it will injure me. The best thing will be for me to vomit it up. Well, now, I will try it. After a few attempts I gave up. I thought to myself, " Well, now you have done it. You have been going around trying everything and now you have done something that has harmed you. What is it ? It seems to be alive and moving in my stomach. If only some of my own people were here ! That would have been better. Now no one will know what has happened to me. I have killed myself " '.[3]

---

[1] 37th A.R.A.B.E., pp. 396-7.   [2] *Op. cit.*, pp. 393-4.
[3] *Op. cit.*, pp. 390 ff.

However, Rave was persuaded to eat peyote again on the second night. They ate ' seven peyote apiece ', whereupon,

> ' Suddenly I saw a big snake. I was very much frightened·
> Then another one came crawling over me. " My God ! where
> are these coming from ? " There at my back there seemed to be
> something. So I looked around and I saw a snake about to
> swallow me entirely. It had legs and arms and a long tail. The
> end of this tail was like a spear. " O, my God ! I am surely
> going to die now," I thought. Then I looked again in another
> direction and I saw a man with horns and long claws and with
> a spear in his hand. He jumped for me and I threw myself on
> the ground. He missed me. Then I looked back and this time
> he started back, but it seemed to me that he was directing his
> spear at me. Again I threw myself on the ground and he missed
> me. There seemed to be no possible escape for me. Then suddenly
> it occurred to me, " Perhaps it is this peyote that is doing this
> thing to me ? " " Help me, O medicine, help me ! It is you who
> are doing this and you are holy ! It is not these frightful visions
> that are causing this. I should have known that you were doing
> it. Help me ! " Then my suffering stopped. " As long as the
> earth shall last, that long will I make use of you, O medicine ! "
> ' This had lasted a night and a day. For a whole night I had
> not slept at all.
> ' Then we breakfasted. Then I said, when we were through,
> " Let us eat peyote again to-night." That evening I ate eight
> peyote.
> ' In the middle of the night I saw God. To God living up above,
> our Father, I prayed : " Have mercy upon me ! Give me know-
> ledge that I may not say and do evil things. To you, O God,
> I am trying to pray. Do thou, O Son of God, help me, too. This
> religion, let me know. Help me, O medicine, grandfather, help
> me ! Let me know this religion ! " Thus I spoke and sat very
> quiet.'

Everything now became good, and a happy vision of his wife appeared.

> ' Indeed, it is good. They are all well—my brother, my sister,
> my father, my mother. I felt very good indeed. O medicine,
> grandfather, most assuredly you are holy ! All that is connected
> with you, that I would like to know and that I would like to
> understand. Help me ! I give myself up to you entirely !
> ' For three days and three nights I had been eating medicine,
> and for three days and three nights I had not slept. Throughout
> all the years that I had lived on earth, I now realized that I had
> never known anything holy. Now, for the first time, I knew it.
> Would that some of the Winnebagoes might also know it ! '[1]

[1] 37th A.R.A.B.E., pp. 390-1.

Dr. Radin comments on this :

> ' To judge from Rave's remarks, his first belief in the peyote had nothing of the nature of a conversion to a new religion. It seems to have been similar to the average Winnebago attitude towards a medicinal plant obtained either as a gift or through purchase. There is only one new note—stimulation by a narcotic.'[1]

Whether we regard Rave's words as indicating ' conversion to a new religion ' or not is largely a matter of how religion is defined. But it does not seem to me to be correct to state that the only new note here is stimulation by a narcotic. The important new note is Rave's remarkable reaction to the effects of that stimulation ; and from the point of view which is being maintained in the present work that reaction has the essential characteristics of religion. That the idea of peyote as the central element in a ' new religion ' in the sense of a definite cult to be established only emerged later is almost certainly true, but that the experience at a very early stage of the peyote eating was definitely religious seems to me beyond dispute. (1) The situation brought about by the effects of peyote eating is entirely baffling : Rave is utterly unable to cope with the intense suffering and affect accompanying the terrible visions. He does not know what to do, and his distress increases in proportion to the intensification of the experience of frustration. (2) At the critical point in this tension an interpretation of the suffering and affect is achieved, which recognizes the visions themselves as effects, not causes. The cry, ' Perhaps it is this peyote that is doing this thing to me ', represents precisely the imaginal interference with an incomprehensible situation which brings it partially within the scope of established modes of response. Peyote at that point ceases to be merely something that can be eaten :

---

[1] *Op. cit.*, p. 419.

it has become something charged with the kind of power with which Rave was conversant through his religious upbringing. (3) Once the situation has undergone this process of interpretation, and the peyote endowed with the quality of ' holiness ', the experience becomes coherent and manageable. Bad visions give place to good ones. Well-being supervenes upon intense distress. And this, of course, is the psychological truth of the interpretation : directly peyote is recognized as an element highly charged with religious power, and is respectfully treated, prayed to, etc., it does good, it heals distress and disease, convicts of sin, and so forth. Here, then, are all the stages of (i) frustration by something utterly beyond the scope of the normally functioning tendencies, (ii) imaginal reconstruction, or interpretation of essential features in the situation, (iii) successful adaptation to the situation, by an acknowledgement that it remains essentially beyond human control, but that it may be induced by ceremonies, faith and other discipline to be favourable.

We are not given any information about the peyote as a religious element previous to its introduction to Rave and its incorporation by him in the new Winnebago Cult. But in a section dealing with ' The Religious Content ' (of the Winnebago Cult) Dr. Radin says :

' We have, of course, first and foremost the peyote. When enough of it has been taken, it acts as a strong stimulant, apparently bringing the nervous system to the highest degree of tension. The pupils of the eyes become dilated, the eyes themselves assume a glazed appearance, while the limbs become rigid. The rhythmic movement of the rattles to the accompaniment of the songs and the drum-beats is quite remarkable for its unison. In short, there are present all the signs of emotional exaltation. This exaltation seems to last until morning. The reaction differs with different individuals ; but in the large majority of cases seems to take the form of a long and profound sleep. Yet I have known quite a number of individuals who did not seem to have any reaction at all.

' What the inner effects are, I know only from description. There seem to be two strongly marked elements ; first, a disagreeable taste, and a choking sensation ; and secondly, a tendency to have visions, generally accompanied by the most gorgeous colour sensations. The visions are always interpreted.

' To judge from John Rave's description of his conversion, he did not interpret the vision initially. He, of course, experienced the choking sensation, and noted the fact that any tendency to struggle against the effects of the peyote accentuated this choking sensation ; while acquiescence relieved it. He seems very early to have associated this struggle with a notion that it was connected with a disbelief in the efficacy of the peyote, and unwillingness to become truly contrite. Later on, he elaborated this into a kind of a dogma—that the disagreeable effects of the peyote varied directly with a man's disbelief in it. This explanation he persistently drummed into the ears of beginners, who might otherwise become terrified and give up too soon. Secondly, he seems to have claimed that the only relief for the sufferer was a formal public declaration of faith in the peyote. To this declaration of faith many details were added by individuals, as they joined the cult, so that gradually it took the stereotyped form of the narration of the former sinful life, magnifying it and announcing the completeness of the change wrought in them by virtue of the peyote. With the exception of these details, there was a definite interpretation of the more immediate effects of the peyote from a rather early time ; and this was followed, with variations, by all new converts.

' The visions were of two kinds ; either they were monsters pursuing an individual, or they constituted more or less elaborate dreams. For the former I found no general interpretation. Each individual was allowed to interpret them or not, as he chose. A number of individuals accepted them as material manifestations of their personal defects of character, one man assuring me that he vomited bulldogs when he first took peyote, and that this symbolized to him deliverance from his bulldog, stubborn nature. The dream visions are interpreted individually, although some are not interpreted at all. For that matter, not all claim to have them. In some cases, the individuals are directed to perform certain actions ; in others, salient facts in their lives are explained '.[1]

The feature of outstanding interest and importance in connection with the peyote is the vision production,

[1] J.R.P., pp. 18-19.

together, of course, with the reaction to the visions. The
fact has already been noted in the preceding chapter that
the Winnebago were in the habit of cultivating dreams and
visions by means of fasting. It may be supposed, therefore, that Rave was not only familiar with the ceremonial
performances of the Winnebago religion, but that he was
conversant with, if he had not enjoyed personal experience
of, the vision effects of fasting. The point is of much
interest.[1] If Rave had already been ' blessed ' by the
spirits through visions in the past, it is not altogether surprising that his experiences after eating peyote should
become, in large measure, assimilated to the earlier and
admittedly religious experiences. If, on the other hand,
Rave had not enjoyed the personal experience of being
' blessed ', but only knew of the experience at second-hand,
we can well understand that suddenly to be plunged into
the experience of vision seeing under the influence of peyote
would bring into operation an attitude of pronounced active
personal faith in place of the passive acquiescence in a
prevailing tradition. What the fasters had proclaimed was
now not only true in the sense that their word might be
believed, but was true in the sense that their experience
was actually duplicated in essential particulars. There are,
nevertheless, elements of novelty or strangeness in the
peyote visions which should be noted. (1) The peyote was
not originally eaten by Rave for any definite religious
purpose, while fasting was undertaken with that end in
view.

' Rave's account of how he first ate peyote tells us nothing of
what induced him to do so. When I put the question to him, he
answered that it was only because of repeated requests '.[2]

[1] See note at end of chapter, p. 117.   [2] J.R.P., p. 8.

That statement, however, is supplemented by another :

> 'Rave's account of his conversion gives a sufficiently dramatic picture of how he first ate the peyote and its immediate effects. In response to numerous questions as to how he was first induced to eat the peyote he always said it was because he had been so frequently asked. It is, however, far more likely that he was passing through an emotional crisis at that particular time, and the requests that he partake of it and the inducements held out to him, made it easier for him to succumb then than on his previous visits '.[2]

If this last suggestion of Dr. Radin's is correct, the motive may have been a religious one, but it still remains unlikely that the motive was to see visions, as was the case in fasting. (2) The initial visions were horrible and harrowing—far from obviously being the vehicles or promises of ' blessing '. The fasting visions bore some resemblance to expectation and desire : it cannot be said that Rave's first peyote visions did the same. (3) The visions were suddenly induced, arriving quite unexpectedly, whereas the fasting visions were often only obtained after a lengthy period and the attainment of a thoroughly ' pitiable ' condition. It is these features which give the character of a new departure to the Cult. . . . Rave stumbles upon an element in reality which has all the characteristics of the ' beyond '— he is in a sense pursued and overtaken by it in the midst of a life of indifference. Peyote, which brings this about, is therefore not to be *identified* with the old religion at any point, though it is obvious that its interpretation is largely conditioned by Rave's knowledge of, and participation in, Winnebago religion. It is ' holy ' on its own account, because, as Rave says, ' it is you who are doing this '— that is, inducing visions and causing suffering.

Undoubtedly the inspiration to react to the suffering

and the horrible visions in the way that Rave did must be attributed in part to what Mr. Bartlett calls a ' religious interest or bent '. What he means by that may be understood by the following passage :

> ' . . . all the available evidence shows us that in Rave's case we have a man whose interests from an early age centre about ceremonial practices. It was not merely that he knew that there were these practices. Every Winnebago would know that. It was not merely that he knew what they were. It was that he had, as Radin says, " participated actively in all the prominent ceremonies ", and had a definite bias in this direction '.

In a footnote to this passage Mr. Bartlett adds :

> ' I may be allowed to point out here that Dr. Radin has seen this interpretation of Rave's character, and has expressed his entire agreement '.[1]

But granting the assumption of a bias or bent as part of the original psychological make-up, we must remember that this means little more than a pre-disposition to form a specific interest if the environment is favourable. I have already suggested that the original bias in the case of Teresa depended for the specificity of its religious direction entirely on environment. And in Rave's case it is clear that his religious interest had been very largely determined not only by participation in prominent ceremonies, but also by familiarity with the fasting experiences, whether he only knew about these, or had enjoyed actual ' blessings '. But his religious interest, thus stimulated and directed by environment, was not limited to any fixed set of phenomena, but was in the nature of an acquired reactive tendency which was ready to function in analogous situations. This is another illustration of the point made in the last chapter : that once established difference tendencies (whether group difference tendencies, or individual difference ten-

[1] *Psychology and Primitive Culture*, p. 175.

dencies) ' overflow ', and help to endow fresh experiences
with a quality of their own.[1] The suffering and bad
visions of the peyote experience are now assimilated by the
interest to the realm of religiously interpreted elements of
reality.   With regard to the evidence for an original bent in
Rave's psychological make-up, I should adduce in addition
to what Bartlett, with Radin's agreement, has said, the
general fact that Rave seems to have been by nature one
of the specially sensitive type, with characteristics of
instability.[2]   This, it has already been suggested, is a native
pre-disposition towards religion, if the environment is
favourable.   Beyond this we hardly have evidence for a
deeper psychological analysis of Rave, and what this
amounts to is that with native plasticity and adaptability,
together with a social environment which encouraged the
direction of his sensitiveness to religion, he was at the time
of eating peyote pre-disposed to discern in his after experiences a religious element.   At the same time it should
be noted that the peyote situation is itself one which may
be regarded as potentially religious without the supposition
of a definite religious interest on the part of the subject
brought into contact with it.   From the point of view of
this book, in so far as all human beings are capable of
discriminating, under certain circumstances, elements in
the environment for dealing with which they have no
specific endowment, they may all be said to have an
' original bent ' in the (probable) direction of religion,
precisely because there are so many points at which the
environment of man has qualities and characteristics which

---

[1] See above, p. 29, p. 65.

[2] The evidence for this has been given in connection with Rave's conversion.   Briefly, the impression is that he was fond of wandering, un-
settled, somewhat loose in habits, subject to ' murderous thoughts.'   See
pp. 96-7 above.   See also note at end of chapter, p. 117.

are unfamiliar and baffling in the absence of a perfectly corresponding and adequate mechanism of response. Peyote, with the effects so vividly described both by Rave and others, undoubtedly possesses such qualities for all people who have not attained the acquired response and comprehension of a scientific attitude, which at once classifies the after effects of peyote eating with other familiar and usual phenomena produced by drugs and narcotics. That is to say, for the unsophisticated person, the peyote feelings and visions represent the invasion of consciousness by a complex of elements for which the person as an agent is wholly unprepared and unequipped.

Bartlett seems inclined to follow Radin in the view that Rave's ' first belief in the peyote had nothing of the nature of a conversion to a new religion '.[1] The question is of crucial importance from the point of view of the present inquiry, and merits further discussion. It may be noted that both Radin and Bartlett write primarily as students of the psychology of borrowing, and by denying that the peyote at the outset had much to do with religion, they are emphasizing the points of similarity in Rave's peyote reactions to those of ordinary Winnebago medicine practice. If they mean to deny that the peyote became a religious object for Rave at the outset, it can only be because they accept a definition of religion which is unduly narrow. What is the evidence ? We have O.L.'s remark to the effect that :

> ' There was not very much religion connected with it in the beginning and the reason people drank it was on account of the peculiar effects it had upon them '[2].

And in addition to Radin's remark already quoted on

---

[1] See note at the end of this chapter, p. 117.   [2] 37th A.R.A.B.E., p. 394.

p. 99, the following passage from the section dealing with *Dissemination of the Doctrine* :

> ' The first and foremost virtue predicated by Rave for the peyote was its curative power. He gives a number of instances in which hopeless venereal diseases and consumption were cured by its use ; and this was the first thing one heard about it as late as 1913. In the early days of the Peyote cult it appears that Rave relied principally for new converts upon the knowledge of this great curative virtue of the peyote. The main point apparently was to induce people to try it. No amount of preaching of its direct effects, such as the hyperstimulation induced, the glorious visions, and the relaxation following, would ever have induced prominent members of the old Winnebago religious societies to try it. For that reason it is highly significant that all the old members of the Peyote cult speak of the diseases of which it cured them. Along this line lay unquestionably its appeal for the most converts. Its subsequent spread was due to a large number of interesting factors. One informant claims that there was little religion connected with it at first, and that the people drank the peyote on account of its peculiar effects '.[1]

But this has to be read in the light of Rave's own very emphatic words about his reaction to the peyote even while he was still enduring intense distress and being persecuted by horrible visions—before, that is, he had experienced anything curative at all. He makes it clear (if we are to trust his account) that it was the sudden realization that peyote was a mysterious agency causing all his sufferings that brought about the change, and led to its beneficent effects. Thus it was not the curative virtue of the peyote which either confirmed Rave's faith or secured that of the converts, but the ' holiness ' of the peyote, expressed, among other ways, in a curative power which was altogether out of the range of common everyday practice, and definitely part of the religious order. Even if the first converts were persuaded to try the new ' medicine ' because of its curative power it does not mean that they were not being

[1] *Op. cit.*, p. 423.

persuaded to embrace a religion. The claim of healing diseases has been in the forefront of many religions, and many persons have been induced to embrace the various religions because they were led to hope for some kind of supernatural healing, not for their spiritual diseases alone, but for their bodily ailments. We have a striking modern instance in the origin and growth of Christian Science. It would hardly be inaccurate description to apply Radin's words, *mutatis mutandis*, quoted overleaf to this most recent of the Christian denominations. The outsider is frequently invited to ' try ' Christian Science, not for the sake of healing a sick soul or saving a lost one, but in order to recover lost health. But to conclude that Christian Science is nothing but a sort of medicine—in our modern sense of the term—would be entirely erroneous. It is essentially religious because it is characterized by an affective, imaginative and intellectual attitude to that which lies beyond the ' natural ' man, and its curative powers are held to be the direct result of a right relationship with this ' beyond ' element, the Unseen Reality, the Divine. While undoubtedly much less reflective and philosophical, the Winnebago attitude is none the less essentially similar. His ' medicine ' throughout is charged with the element of mystery, and the shamanistic practices contain within them the essentials of religion no less than the practices of the so-called religious societies. Concerning Shamanistic and Medicinal Practices, Radin says :

' The Winnebago make a fourfold classification of their medicines. Those that affect a person by direct administration ; those that affect him by odour, like love and racing medicines ; those that affect him at a distance ; and those that are shot at an individual. Most of the medicines are obtained by fasting, although they can also be bought. . . .

'Medicine may be used in a number of ways, but principally as offerings or as means of killing animals or men '.[1]

In the account of *How An Indian Shaman Cures His Patients* the religious nature of medicines and medicinal practices is very clearly brought out.

'I came from above and I am holy (says the shaman). . . . Once when I was on the warpath I was killed. It seemed to me, however, as if I had merely stumbled '.[2]

After many transformations he was permitted to go to his ' higher spirit-home ', where he was ' blessed ' by all the spirits, after appropriate fastings. So effective were those ' blessings ' that

'I can dictate to all the spirits that exist. Whatever I say will come to pass. The tobacco you (the patients) offer me is not to be used by myself. It is really intended for the spirits '.[3]

The treatment of the patient then consists mainly in making offerings of tobacco to the various spirits, with an appropriate prayer, consisting of a reminder of promises received from them in ' blessings '—forms of prayer which, changing the name of the spirit addressed, and one or two other local details, can be heard in almost any church. It is abundantly clear that the healing is dependent upon the incalculable power of the spirits, which can to some extent be made available for human ends by the shaman through getting into right relations with the spirits. The fact is that it is, as Dr. W. H. R. Rivers has shewn, quite a late development of thought and insight which distinguishes ' medicine, magic and religion ' one from the other. Primarily the reaction to what we to-day distinguish as three separate realms is identical :

---

[1] 37th A.R.A.B.E., p. 254. [2] *Op. cit.*, p. 270.
[3] *Op. cit.*, p. 272.

' Among ourselves (Rivers writes) these three groups of process are more or less sharply marked off from one another. One has gone altogether into the background of our social life, while the other two form distinct social categories widely different from one another, and having few elements in common. If we survey mankind widely this distinction and separation do not exist. There are many peoples among whom the three sets of social process are so closely inter-related that the disentanglement of each from the rest is difficult or impossible '.[1]

Again the same writer says :

' The great majority of the measures by which existing savage peoples attempt to cope with disease fall into one or other of the two categories of religion and magic '.[2]

It cannot be too strongly emphasized that, convenient as it is for us to distinguish ' magic ' from ' religion ', there is no essential difference from the point of view of the psychological mechanisms involved : a fact already dealt with both directly and by implication.[3] In precisely the same

---

[1] *Medicine, Magic, and Religion*, 1924, p. 1.   [2] *Op. cit.*, p. 120.
[3] See above, chapters I and II. E. B. Tylor treated the distinction between Religion and ' Occult Science and Magic ' as fundamental. Religion, he asserts (*Primitive Culture*, 4th ed., vol. i, p. 424) is based on ' the belief in Spiritual beings,' while Occult Science and Magic arise from an erroneous application of the association of ideas (vol. i, p. 116). Sir J. G. Frazer's view is similar. Religion is ' a propitiation or conciliation of powers superior to man which are believed to direct and control the course of nature and of human life,' while magic is based on a sort of pseudo-science : ' Its fundamental conception is identical with that of modern science ; underlying the whole system is a faith, implicit but real and firm, in the order and uniformity of nature.' (*The Golden Bough*, vol. i, p.p. 220, 222). Westermarck, again, is in agreement : ' Religion may be defined as a belief in and a regardful attitude towards a supernatural being on whom man feels himself dependent and to whose will he makes appeal in his worship.' But ' the supernatural, like the natural, may be looked upon in the light of mechanical energy, which discharges itself without the aid of any volitional activity,' and it is this which constitutes magic. ' He who performs a purely magical act utilizes such power without making any appeal at all to the will of a supernatural being.' (*The Origin and Development of the Moral Ideas*, 1908, vol. ii, p. 584). The distinction is a useful one for purposes of classification, but it is a distinction *within* the realm of religious phenomena, and not *between* the religious and something other. Rivers, with his special psychological qualifications, recognized this, though still finding the distinction useful. ' The distinction between magic and religion,' he says, *Medicine, Magic and Religion*, p. 3, ' is one which has long tried the ingenuity of students of human society. Among many peoples, including those with whom this book will especially deal, it is far from easy to draw any definite

way, until medicine has entered upon its modern phase, it is psychologically a specific department of what is generically Religion. To quote Rivers again :

line between the two, and we need a term which will include both.' In an unpublished paper of my own, written 1912, *The Significance of the Religious Consciousness for Epistemology*, I wrote : ' Is the distinction between Magic and Religion, so clearly drawn by Westermarck, in common with other anthropological writers, of any other significance than a classificatory one ? Is not the impulse which finds expression in what is called religion precisely the same as that which finds expression in magic ? Religion may be partially characterized, but not defined, as *the expression of a desire to get some knowledge of and control over the uncertainties of life*. The impulse which renders man restless in time of drought until he can do or say something to bring about rain is one form of the religious impulse : for the making of rain is beyond the control of ordinary men and requires special means to be adopted. That impulse of man to make himself at home among the uncertainties of life finds expression in what Westermarck calls Magic as well as in what he calls Religion : the impulse is one and is the basal impulse of all religious striving and construction. We might retain the conventional classification, while recognizing the underlying unity of the religious impulse thus :

Religious Impulse

Magical Religion	Personal Religion

We shall then mean by Magical Religion what Westermarck means by Magic, and by Personal Religion what he means by Religion.' R. R. Marett takes a point of view on this particular matter with which the present book is in entire agreement. The following passages are taken from *The Threshold of Religion*, 2nd ed. 1914. ' . . . if there is reason, as I think there is, to hold that man's religious sense is a constant and universal feature of his mental life, its essence and true nature must then be sought, not so much in the shifting variety of its ideal constructions, as in that steadfast groundwork of specific emotion whereby man is able to feel the supernatural precisely at the point at which his thought breaks down.' (p. 28) ' I do not find that the leading theorists have by the organization of their material shown themselves to be sufficiently aware that the animistic idea represents but one amongst a number of ideas, for the most part far more vague than it is, and hence more liable to escape notice ; all of which ideas, however, are active in savage religion as we have it, struggling one with the other for supremacy in accordance with the normal tendency of religious thought towards uniformity of doctrinal expression.' (p. 26-7) ' First, I suppose certain beliefs, of a kind natural to the infancy of thought, to be accepted at face value in a spirit of naive faith, whilst being in fact illusory. The practice corresponding to such naive belief I call " rudimentary magic '. Afterwards I conceive a certain sense of their *prima facie* illusiveness to come to attach to these beliefs, without, however, managing to invalidate them. This I call the stage of " developed magic ". Such magic, as embodying a reality that to some extent transcends appearance, becomes to a corresponding extent a mystery. As such, on my view, it tends to fall within the sphere of religion. For I define the object of religion to be whatever is perceived as a mystery and treated accordingly.' (pp. 32-3)

' Medicine . . . is a term for a set of social practices by which man seeks to direct and control a specific group of natural phenomena, viz., those especially affecting man himself, which so influence his behaviour as to unfit him for the normal accomplishment of his physical and social functions—phenomena which lower his vitality and tend towards death. By a process of generalization, society has come to classify these phenomena together, and has distinguished them from other groups of natural phenomena under the name of disease '.[1]

Just so long as this specific group of phenomena is reacted to by man as having the character of the mysterious, or the ' beyond ', his practices in relation to them, though we may describe them as ' medicine ' or as ' magic ' are actually religious.

It seems clear, then, that the mere curative value of the peyote was not the primary element in it for Rave or for any of his converts. Even leaving aside the statement Rave makes that he had recognized it as ' holy ' even while it was making him bad, and not curing him at all, and supposing it to have been its beneficent effects that really established his view of its ' holiness ', it still remains indisputable that it is *the curative effects of something which is holy*, a curative virtue which works in ways not to be identified with the ordinary, which occupies the centre of the picture. It is, in a word, the disparateness felt between human power and expectation, and the actual effects of the peyote, which is constitutive of the cult. Religion comes into being at the point where human faculties are frustrated.

Nevertheless, I think that the curative qualities of the peyote, even so understood, are given by Radin a more prominent place in the establishment of the cult than the evidence warrants. The outstanding features, as already

---

[1] *Medicine, Magic and Religion* , pp. 4-5.

indicated, are the intense affect and the induction of a trance-like condition, usually accompanied by visions. In Rave's own case it seems to have been a combination of the terribly intense suffering and the vivid and horrible visions that prepared the way for his attribution of ' holiness ' to the peyote. The fact that he was cured of a disease is only mentioned later on in his narrative, as an item in a whole list of benefits received *when once the religious response to the peyote and its effects had been initiated.* The same thing is strikingly illustrated in J.B.'s Peyote Experiences. This is a long, but extremely interesting and important narrative, in the course of which the author of it reveals several marked traits—as for instance extreme suggestibility, and sexual susceptibility and activity. The story is too lengthy to reproduce in full, but the following summary may suffice. J.B. was at first prejudiced against the peyote and peyote eaters, and his prejudice was reinforced by the express injunction of his youngest sister— ' the one to whom we always listened most attentively '— and he promised her he would not eat peyote. However, other relatives among whom he went to stay were peyote eaters, and they and other members of the cult combined to treat J.B. with the utmost kindness, consideration and tenderness. He fenced with them at first, however, though he was not above pretending to be more sympathetic than in fact he was, for sake of obliging his friends :

' At night they had their ceremony. At first I sat outside and listened to them. I was rather fond of them. I stayed in that country and the young peyote eaters were exceedingly friendly to me. They would give me a little money now and then, and they treated me with tender regard. They did everything that they thought would make me feel good, and in consequence I used to speak as though I liked their ceremony. However, I was only deceiving them. I only said it because they were so good to me.

I thought they acted in this way because (the peyote) was deceiving them '.[1]

He even went so far as to disobey his youngest sister's injunction, and ate peyote, and stood up in the meeting at the request of his brother-in-law and ' younger ' sister to ' give himself up ', but there was still nothing in the nature of a conversion :

> ' I did not like it, but I did it nevertheless. " Why should I give myself up ? I am not in earnest, and I intend to stop this as soon as I get back to Wisconsin. I am only doing this because they have given me presents," I thought. " I might just as well get up, since it doesn't mean anything to me ". So I stood up '.[2]

But then he began to feel sick, and lost consciousness, and on recovery he was vexed that he had eaten peyote :

> ' " Why have I done this ? " I said to myself. " I promised (my sister) that I would not do it ". So I thought and then I tried to leave, but I could not. I suffered intensely. At last daylight came upon me. Now I thought that they regarded me as one who had a trance and found out something '.[3]

After this he suffered the peyote people to cut off his hair and to take from him much medicine that he had—many small bundles of ' courting medicine '—but even after these articles had been burnt, and after he had been assured that he understood (which pleased him), he still admits that

> ' (As a matter of fact) I had not received any knowledge '.[4]

The crucial experience, however, eventually came at a later meeting, when he ate ' a lot of peyote ' :

> ' It was now late at night and I had eaten a lot of peyote and felt rather tired. I suffered considerably. After a while I looked at the peyote and there stood an eagle with outspread wings. It was as beautiful a sight as one could behold. Each of the feathers seemed to have a mark. The eagle stood looking at me. I looked around thinking that perhaps there was something the matter with my sight. Then I looked again and it was really

[1] 37th A.R.A.B.E., p. 401.   [2] *Op. cit.*, p. 405.   [3] *Op. cit.*, p. 405.
[4] *Op. cit.*, p. 406.

there. I then looked in a different direction and it disappeared. Only the small peyote remained. I looked around at the other people but they all had their heads bowed and were singing. I was very much surprised.

' Some time after this (I saw) a lion lying in the same place (where I had seen the eagle). I watched it very closely. It was alive and looking at me. I looked at it very closely, and when I turned my eyes away just the least little bit it disappeared. " I suppose they all know this and I am just beginning to know of it," I thought. Then I saw a small person (at the same place). He wore blue clothes and a shining brimmed cap. He had on a soldier's uniform. He was sitting on the arm of the person who was drumming, and he looked at every one. He was a little man, perfect (in all proportions). Finally I lost sight of him. I was very much surprised indeed. I sat very quietly, " This is what it is ", I thought, " this is what they all probably see and I am just beginning to find out ".

' Then I prayed to Earthmaker (God) : " This, your ceremony, let me hereafter perform ".

' As I looked again I saw a flag. I looked more carefully and (I saw) the house full of flags. They had the most beautiful marks on them. In the middle (of the room) there was a very large flag and it was a live one ; it was moving. In the doorway there was another one not entirely visible. I had never seen anything so beautiful in all my life before.

' Then again I prayed to Earthmaker (God) I bowed my head and closed my eyes and began (to speak). I said many things that I would ordinarily never have spoken about. As I prayed, I was aware of something above me and there he was ; Earthmaker (God) to whom I was praying, he it was. That which is called the soul, that is it, that is what one calls Earthmaker (God). Now this is what I felt and saw. All of us sitting there, we had all together one spirit or soul ; at least that is what I learned. I instantly became the spirit and I was their spirit or soul. Whatever they thought of, I (immediately) knew. I did not have to speak to them and get an answer to know what their thoughts had been. Then I thought of a certain place, far away, and immediately I was there ; I was my thought '.[1]

Throughout this narrative the curative qualities of the peyote are only mentioned once, and that by J.B.'s father, in giving a preliminary account (and by no means a wholly favourable one) of the peyote people. He said :

' " It does not amount to anything, all this that they are doing, although they do stop drinking. It is also said that sick people

[1] *Op. cit.*, pp. 406-7.

get well. We were told about this and so we joined, and, sure enough, we are practically well, your mother as well as I " '.[1]

But it does not anywhere appear that it was a desire to get well that induced J.B. himself to eat peyote : what prevailed upon him, apparently, was, in the first instance, social pressure, and more particularly the influence of relatives. But his being induced to eat the peyote did not at first bring about a conversion experience : what achieved this was, once again, visions after an intense feeling of suffering. Through these visions he came into direct contact with the mysterious, the something beyond normal expectation, which overwhelmed his scepticism in the very process of defeating all his established modes of response. The whole story gives point to Rave's remark, towards the close of his own narrative :

> ' If you just hear about it you are not likely to try it. If you desire real knowledge about it try it yourself, for then you will learn of things that you had never known before '.[2]

In a word, the peyote is holy, for it introduces man to mysterious and tremendous power, utterly beyond his understanding ; if this power is not accepted and believed in, it can and will cause terrible suffering, but if surrender is made to it, and an attitude of faith adopted, it will bestow all manner of blessings, of which one is the healing of disease.

[1] 37th A.R.A.B.E., p. 401.   [2] *Op. cit.*, p. 393.

NOTE ADDED TO CHAPTERS III AND IV

I am permitted by Dr. Radin, who has very kindly read the two chapters on ' The Religion of the Winnebago ' and ' The Peyote Cult Among the Winnebago ', to say that he is in entire agreement with the interpretation of the Winnebago material set forth in these two chapters, including the one or two passages in which I have offered some criticism of his presentation and conclusions. The most important of these is on p. 106 ff.

Regarding the question raised on p. 102, Dr. Radin tells me that Rave did not obtain a ' blessing '. He seems to have lacked the stability of purpose to continue the fasting experience long enough to ensure the induction of visions. I may also add, concerning the reference on p. 105 to Rave's ' instability ', that Dr. Radin fully endorses what I have said.

V

GEORGE FOX

IF Radin's account of the introduction of the Peyote Cult among the Winnebago Indians affords us an instructive instance of the effects of frustration and an expansion of consciousness, leading to a religious experience at a simple level of culture, the Journal of George Fox provides us with an equally illuminating example in a more complex civilization. Moreover, in this instance, we have the advantage of a much fuller autobiography, together with the comments and interpretations of several other writers. There is here, no less than in the case of the Peyote Cult, a fruitful field for the student of the psychology of borrowing ; but this aspect of the subject will be entirely subordinated here, as in the last chapter, to the specifically religious question. From the point of view of my present interest, the problem is neither one which has to do with the definite and conscious introduction of new religious ideas into an established culture, nor the conscious welding together of various elements of religious belief and behaviour derived from the environment. Fox is, above all, the founder of Quakerism, which, however similar it may be to other religious movements of the time, was quite definitely a new growth around the personality and teaching of Fox ; and his indebtedness to other movements was due almost certainly not to any conscious borrowing, but to the unconscious influences of suggestion.

Hodgkin may perhaps emphasize too strongly the originality of Fox, on the ground of his ' knowing scarce any other
book than the English Bible ',[1] but there is no evidence of
conscious borrowing. Ideas which have been sown in the
mind by suggestion often emerge into consciousness with
all the characteristics of freshness and novelty. The
problem here to be dealt with is primarily Fox's own
religious experience and response, and for the adequate
analysis of this we need to take into account, at least
briefly, the general background of the situation, social and
religious, as it existed in England at the time, as well as
Fox's own psychological make-up.

George Fox was born at the close of the reign of James I,
and his childhood and early youth were spent in the
troublous times of Charles I. The period was one of great
religious and political unrest, maturing rapidly for the
upheaval of the Civil War. And to a large extent the
religious and political forces of unrest were the same.
Puritanism, as it found expression in Cromwell and the
Commonwealth, was an attempt to make the politics of
England conformable to the politics of a kingdom of God
on earth, as then understood and interpreted. Law,
justice, and the sword were all regarded as instruments
for this ' settlement ' of England, which was to be equally
political and religious. Nor was the other main branch
of Puritanism less political. Presbyterianism, though in
conflict with the tyranny of kingship and that of episcopalianism, had no conception of a separation of religion and
state, but aimed at replacing the uniformity of the old

[1] Thomas Hodgkin, *George Fox*, 1896, p. 2. It is interesting to compare
with this the statement of Dr. Rachel Knight, *The Founder of Quakerism*,
The Swarthmore Press, 1922, on p. 155, in connection with the writings
of Boehme : ' Undoubtedly Fox read them. It was his custom to read
many books, and to carry other books than the Bible with him.'

system by a compulsory uniformity of its own. Thus although the period is usually regarded as being one of intense religious ferment—and it undoubtedly was a period of ferment *about* religion—it was in the main a ferment around externals, forms, privileges, government and creeds, rather than about the *fundamentals of experience*. There seems to have been more concern about the form and government of the Church, and the orthodoxy of its creeds, among the people generally, than of concern about the religious content of the Christian Gospel. Thus Robert Barclay says :

' When the sanction of Parliament was asked in 1571 to the Thirty-nine Articles of the Church of England (which were in January, 1562-3, only agreed upon by convocation without alteration in a Puritan sense by a majority of *one vote*), the House of Commons declined to adopt the thirty-sixth and the other articles relating to the hierarchy and ritual of the Church. This shews the purely political character of the Puritan movement. It concerned the things of religion, but it remained from this period to the accession of Charles II., true to the one idea of substituting by constitutional means, a Presbyterian form of State Church for the Anglican '.[1]

The Civil War, which broke out in 1642, when Fox was eighteen, was the inevitable outcome of the seething conflict of political and religious opinions and convictions. Its issue—from the point of view of religion—was largely to make explicit many things which had been implicit in the severance of the English Church from Rome. What that severance actually involved was a rejection of the claims of ecclesiasticism to be the sole depository and interpreter of truth. As it was the English Bible that largely overthrew Roman Catholicism in England, the upholders of the Reformed Church speedily took refuge in the authority of Scripture as the only bulwark against papal supremacy,

[1] *The Inner Life of the Religious Societies of the Commonwealth*, 1876, pp. 14-15.

and thus the seat of authority, hitherto recognized as the Catholic Church, now became the Bible. But without the authorized ecclesiastical interpretation of the Bible, its words could provide no universally agreed standard of theology or of Church government. Only by a dogmatic and fixed interpretation on the part of Protestantism could the Bible become the basis of religious uniformity—as Luther[1] and Calvin[2] clearly recognized. But in this

---

[1] Of Luther, J. R. Green, in *A Short History of the English People*, 1878, p. 315, says : 'From the golden dream of a new age, wrought peaceably and purely by the slow progress of intelligence, the growth of letters, the development of human virtue, the Reformer of Wittenberg turned away with horror. He had little or no sympathy with the new culture. He despised reason as heartily as any Papal dogmatist could despise it. He hated the very thought of toleration or comprehension. He had been driven by a moral and intellectual compulsion to declare the Roman system a false one, but it was only to replace it by another system of doctrine just as elaborate, and claiming precisely the same infallibility.'

[2] Of Calvin, Robert Barclay, *op. cit.*, pp. 16-17, says : ' According to Calvin the whole body of the people were the Church ; where two or three were gathered together there was a Church ; but the system of Calvin eliminated the *voluntary* consent of the two or the three thus gathering, and forced, under heavy penalties, the ungodly and the unbeliever into the Church. The officers of the Church were Ministers, Doctors, or Teachers, Lay-Elders, and Deacons, who formed the Consistory or Church government. The people were admitted to the right of exercising a veto upon the appointment of officers. The Church was co-extensive with the State because it embodied every citizen, and every citizen was subject to the discipline of the Consistory. The censures of the Church were carried out by the sword of the State. The constitution of the theocracy established by Calvin, embodied in its most perfect form, the union of the Church and State, and it is one of the most curious studies in history. Calvin's object was to found a state resembling that of the Israelites under Moses, and the result was one of the most fearful ecclesiastical tyrannies to which mankind has been subjected. The discipline of the Church was carried out with a severity in which the gentle influences of Christianity can hardly be traced. Spies or watchmen were appointed to report even the conversation of the citizens, and the Consistory had power to examine all the citizens, without respect of persons, on the tenderest point of conscience. To impugn Calvin's doctrine or the proceedings of the consistory, subjected persons to banishment on pain of death. The well-known case of Servetus, a learned physician of Unitarian views, simply illustrates the ordinary features of the theocratic government founded by Calvin, carried out to their extreme results. He escaped from the prison of the Inquisition only to be burnt alive at Geneva.' And on p. 18 : ' The power of Calvin's system over that of any previous Protestant reformer's, consisted in a greater logical consistency. It freed Protestantism from all dependence upon human tradition. It sought to bring every sphere of life under the rigid rule of a Church which claimed exclusive possession of the truth, and was prepared to maintain its position in the field of argument.'

respect the Puritans were by no means in agreement among themselves. Many of the leaders of the Long Parliament, such as Pym himself, were in favour of Episcopalianism, and only tended towards Presbyterianism under the pressure of circumstances,[1] while in the army the cream of Cromwell's men were 'sectaries' of various sorts who claimed, no less than the Presbyterians or Episcopalians, the authority of the Bible for their faith and church order. The logical outcome of the break with Rome was, in fact, religious freedom and toleration—a fact which could only be appreciated in a psychological atmosphere less charged with passion than that of the Civil War and Commonwealth period. The idea of toleration received scant attention, and the result was a strife of the sects which became the more vehement and embittered as the primary aim of Puritanism seemed to have been secured by the overthrow of the king, and later by his execution. Indeed, the execution of the king was instrumental in fomenting the hostility between the Independents and 'sectaries' on the one hand, and the more conservative reformers, Presbyterian and Episcopalian, on the other.

What characterizes the period of the Commonwealth from the religious side more, perhaps, than anything else,

---

[1] J. R. Green, *op. cit.*, p. 543 : ' It was with strictly conservative aims in ecclesiastical as in political matters that Pym and his colleagues began the strife. Their avowed purpose was simply to restore the Church of England to its state under Elizabeth, and to free it from innovations, from the changes introduced by Laud and his fellow prelates. The great majority of the Parliament were averse to any alterations in the constitution or doctrine of the Church itself ; and it was only the refusal of the bishops to accept any diminution of their power and revenues, the growth of a party hostile to Episcopalian Government, the necessity for purchasing the aid of the Scots by a union in religion as in politics, and above all the urgent need of constructing some new ecclesiastical organization in the place of the older organization which had become impossible from the Royalist attitude of the bishops, that forced on the two Houses the adoption of the Covenant.' And p. 454 : ' Pym and Hampden had no sort of objection to episcopacy.'

is the astonishing interest which was popularly shewn in questions of doctrine and church organization. Principal Graham says :

> ' The nation's interests and controversies at that time were in the main religious. When George Fox was born the emancipation from Rome was only as far away as the Corn Laws are from us. His mother indeed was " of the stock of the martyrs ". Popery, prelacy, presbytery, and a host of minor systems and doctrines, struggled for souls. Sermons were events as important as cricket matches are now ; and Calvinism and Arminianism were debated as hotly as the Capital Levy '.[1]

William C. Braithwaite is even more specific :

> . . . on the doctrinal side, religion exerted triumphant authority. The episcopal system had disappeared for the time with its votaries, without leaving a great void in the hearts of the nation, because the current Calvinism of the day had become the religion of the people, and it mattered little whether it came from the lips of an Episcopalian or Presbyterian or Baptist divine. Laud had appealed indeed, from the dogmatism of Puritanism to the cultivated intelligence for the solution of religious problems ; but those whom he reached were in exile, and the multitude regarded religion as a thing of doctrinal profession. The authority of doctrine, or what the first Friends called " notions ", held sway as it has not done in England before or since. In the first half of the seventeenth century men seemed under a compulsion to construct a scheme of Divine truth which should satisfy the intellect. The new translations of the Bible had fertilized the world with Bible knowledge and given many an education in religious things which, in the zest of the fresh study, seemed to make them masters of Divine truth. The Bible was regarded as the one authoritative Word of God, which contained a full provision of infallible truth, and doctrinal theology became every man's occupation. . . . This general knowledge of the Bible was now diffused, and accordingly when the era passed in which the State repressed schisms and sects, it was at once succeeded by an age of controversial warfare between conflicting opinions. Polemic replaced persecution, and its virulence was at least better than the fires of Smithfield. In the keen doctrinal atmosphere of the time, a day's dispute in public between opposing combatants was the most delightful and improving of pastimes. A Puritan divine, for example, at Henley-in-Arden, would take up the cudgels against preaching without a call and argue his case with

[1] Article, *Hibbert Journal*, vol. XXII., No. 4 (July, 1924), pp. 689-90.

five private preachers—a nailer, a baker, a plough-wright, a weaver, and a baker's boy. When Thomas Taylor, who afterwards became a Friend, disputed at Kendal, in 1650, on the subject of infant-baptism in the parish church against three other ministers, and had got the better of them, his hearers ran up Kendal Street crying, " Mr. Taylor hath got the day ! Mr. Taylor hath got the day ! " with an enthusiasm now reserved for the result of a game of football '.[1]

Nevertheless it would be a mistake to suppose that the religious interest was solely of this doctrinal and external character. Among the crowd of warring sects which had sprung into existence before or during the Commonwealth[2] we hear of groups of men and women who are dissatisfied with the dogmatism and externalism of all religious parties, and who withdraw to prepare themselves for fuller light and faith. These were the ' Seekers ', who played a very important part in the first spread of the Quaker movement. Concerning the Seekers Barclay says :

' . . . it is certain that the " Seekers " are mentioned by name, as a religious body or party, by Morton, one of the first English Mennonite or General Baptist writers, as early as the year 1617. . . . Saltmarsh gives a clear account of the views of the " Seekers ". He says that they " find that the Christians of the first or Apostles' time . . . were men visibly and spiritually endowed with power from on high, or with the gifts of the Spirit, and so were able to make clear and evident demonstration of God amongst them, as in the churches of all the Christians then in Corinth, Ephesus ", etc. ; and " that all who administered in any outward office as to spiritual things were visibly gifted ". There was *then* an " apostle, evangelist, prophet ", etc., etc., and " all administered in the anointing or unction of Spirit, clearly, certainly, infallibly ; they ministered as the oracles of God. But now, in this time of the apostacy of the churches, they find no such gifts, and so dare not preach, baptise, or teach, etc., or have any church fellowship, because they find no attainment yet in any churches, or church ways, or administration of ordinances,

---

[1] *The Beginnings of Quakerism*, 1912, pp. 16-18.
[2] J. R. Green, *op. cit.*, p. 544, says : ' Four years after the war had begun a horror-stricken pamphleteer numbered sixteen religious sects as existing in defiance of the law ; and, widely as these bodies differed among themselves, all (were ?) at one in repudiating any right of control in faith or worship by the Church or its clergy.'

according to the pattern of the New Testament, etc., etc. There-fore they *wait* in this time of the apostacy of the church ; they *wait*, only in prayer and conference ". They wait for an apostle, or angel, able in the spirit to give some visible demonstration of their sending, etc. . . . It is obvious that among the " Seekers " there was a strong mystical tendency. Cromwell, in his letter to his daughter, Bridget Ireton, written in 1646, tells her that her sister Claypole is " exercised with some perplexed thoughts . . . to be a Seeker is to be of the best sect next to a finder ". . . . John Jackson, one of the Seekers, gives the following explaration of the views and practices of the middle or more moderate class of Seekers. Firstly, they seek the mind of God in the Scriptures. Secondly, they judge that prayer and alms are to be attended to, and for this purpose they come together " into some place on the First-days as their hearts are drawn forth and opportunity offers ". They then seek " firstly, that they may be instruments in the hand of the Lord to stir up the grace of God in one another, by mutual conference and communication of experience ". Second-ly, to wait for a further revelation. Thirdly, to hold out their " testimony against the false, and for the pure ordinance of ministry and worship ". They behave themselves as persons who have neither " the power nor the gift to go before one another by way of eminency, or authority, but as sheep unfolded, and as soldiers unrallied, waiting for a time of gathering ", etc. They acknowledge " no other visible teacher but the Word and Works of God, on whom they wait, for the grace which is to be brought at the revelation of Jesus Christ. . . .''

' We smile when we read of " Seekers ", but the very name expresses a great fact in the spiritual history of this nation. In those days men's hearts were stirred to their very depths. Thous-ands felt that they needed something more than the empty show of religion. They wished to grasp the reality. It is fancied by some that the mere fashion of the times will account for sermons of two or three hours, and prayers of an hour long being listened to with rapt attention, but it was not so. There is every evidence that the strongest heads believed, and the stoutest hearts were bowed under the conviction, that an offended God was pleading with a nation who had deeply transgressed His holy laws. The splendid imagery of the Jewish prophets and the Book of Revela-tions was applied to the state of the nation, and there were few who did not expect that some extraordinary era was about to commence '.[1]

Nor were the Seekers the only groups of people who were concerned about the inner and fundamental realities of religious experience. It is most probable, as R. M. Jones

[1] Robert Barclay, *op. cit.*, pp. 175-6 and 181-2.

and W. C. Braithwaite indicate, that Fox was unconsciously indebted to other influences of a mystical and semi-mystical kind which were being spread abroad in England about this time.[1] While the multitude found ample scope for the exercise of their active tendencies in political partizanship and controversy about the forms and doctrines of religion, culminating in the actual conflict of the civil war, there were individuals and groups here and there who seem to have found no adequate outlet for their tendencies in the characteristic and prevailing fashion, because they were dimly aware of, and profoundly affected by, something in the total situation which could not be thus dealt with. Of the groups perhaps the most striking were the Familists, or Family of Love, which originated, according to Braithwaite, ' about 1530 ', in Holland. Robert Barclay states that Henry Nicholas or Niclaes

> ' founded this extraordinary secret religious Society between the years 1541 and 1590 '.[2]

It seems to have flourished in England for about a century, disappearing about the time of the Commonwealth, as Barclay says :

> ' in the fierce and open struggle of the time between truth and error '.[3]

Two further quotations from this writer will serve to indicate the general character of this group :

> ' They presented a supplication to James I. which was published at Cambridge, 1606, in which they complain that many of them have been cast into prison, and beg the king to judge of them by the Christian rule : " Ye shall know a tree by its fruits ". They say they utterly disclaim and detest all the disobedient and erroneous sects of the Anabaptists, the Brownists, the followers of Penrie, the Puritans, etc., and that his Majesty is under a great

---

[1] Barclay, apparently, considered that Fox was consciously indebted to some of them, notably to the followers of Boehme. See below, p. 127-9.
[2] Robert Barclay, *op. cit.*, p. 26.   [3] *Op. cit.*, p. 32.

misapprehension of them. With the Puritans they say they
" have nothing in common ". . . . They agree with all the Holy
Scriptures as we do understand them. The end of all Henry
Nichclas's writings, say they, is " that all people, when they hear,
read, and do perceive their sins estranging from God and Christ,
might bring forth fruits of repentance and newness of life, açcording
as the Holy Scriptures require of every one, and that they might
in that sort become saved through Jesus Christ, the only Saviour
of the world ". . . .

' The whole of the movements of the Society which Nicholas
founded, were conducted with the utmost secrecy. They have,
however, received a full elucidation in two manuscripts discovered
at Leyden, and the revelation which they furnish of the elaborate
hierarchy which this enthusiast attempted to perpetuate, proves
that his sympathies lay with Roman Catholics, and that, on the
belief in an extraordinary revelation made to himself, he attempted
to spiritualize and to fulfil what he deemed to be the hidden
meaning of the Roman Catholic church, and to found a new society.
His idea being, that the last and final dispensation was the perfect
union of humanity with God, expressed by " Love ", as the
highest state of Christian perfection '.[1]

Of the individual influences of a mystical character which
must have affected Fox either directly or indirectly, the
most important is that of Jacob Boehme. The external
similarities between the shoe-maker of Goerlitz and Fox
in the matter of condition and mode of experience are
striking enough, but more striking are the similarities of
view and of expression given in writing to experiences.
Barclay considers that there are all the evidences that Fox

' had a thorough knowledge of the ideas current in his times,
and the mere perusal of the titles of his tracts will show that he
kept himself abreast of the great questions which agitated the
public mind, and which are expressed in the controversial and
other religious literature of the day '.

and he gives the following quotations in parallel columns
from the writings of Boehme and Fox as convincing
evidence that

' not only was Fox conversant with Boehmen's writings, but
appears in his journal to presuppose a knowledge of Boehmen's
method of stating spiritual experience '.

[1] Robert Barclay, *op. cit.*, pp. 26-27 and p. 30.

FOX

BOEHMEN

' " The second Book concerning the three Principles of the Divine Essence—of the Eternal Dark, Light and Temporary World, showing what the Soul, the Image and the Spirit of the Soul are; also what Angels, Heaven, and Paradise are; how Adam was *before* the Fall, *in* the Fall, and *after* the Fall ", etc., by Jacob Behmen, alias Teutonicus Philosophus, London, 1641 '.

' " Now I was come up in spirit *through the Flaming Sword* into the paradise of God, all things were new ; and all the creation gave another smell unto me than before beyond what words can utter. I knew nothing but pureness, innocency and righteousness, being renewed up into the image of God by Jesus Christ, so that I was come up to the state of Adam before he fell.

' " . . . . then he let them out of the garden, and set the cherubim with a naked (or warning flaming sword) . . . before it to keep the way to the Tree of Life. . . . But the understanding of us poor children of Adam and Eve is sunk so much, that at our last old age we scarce reach the understanding of anything concerning the Fall of Adam and Eve, seeing we must seek very deep for it in the Light of Life, for it is very wonderful which Moses saith, ' God set the cherubim before the garden to keep and guard the way to the Tree of Life ', who could understand it ? If God did not open our eyes, we should speak simply of a Keeper with a sword, and Reason seeth nothing else, but the Noble Virgin showeth us the Door, and *now we must enter into paradise through* the sharpness of the sword, yet the sword cutteth the *Earthly* body clean away from the *Holy Element*, and then the *new man* may enter into paradise by the way of life. . . . Now if anybody would come into the Garden, he must

' " The Creation was opened to me—how all things had their names given them, according to their nature and virtue. I was at a stand in my mind whether I should practise physic for the good of mankind, seeing the nature and virtues of the creatures were opened to me by the Lord " '.

press in *through* the Sword of Death—though Christ hath broken the Sword, so that now we can much easier enter *in with our Souls*, yet *there is a Sword before it still* " '.

' XIII. " After this, about the year 1600, in the 25th year of his age, he was again surrounded with the Divine Life, and replenished with the Heavenly knowledge, in so much as going abroad into the fields, into a green before Neysgate, at Gorlitz, he then sat down, and viewing the Herbs and Grass of the Field in his Inward Light, he saw into their essences use and properties, which were discovered to him by their linaments, figures, and signatures ". Behmen's *Signatura Rerum* was published in English, 1649.—*Life of Jacob Behmen*, by W. Law, London, 1764.

' It can hardly be contended that this, which is one of the most curious and unintelligible passages in Fox's Journal, was written by a person who had never read Behmen's works, which had at that period a considerable circulation '.[1]

This view of direct, if not conscious, borrowing on the part of Fox is in striking opposition to that of Hodgkin, who says :

' . . . the future Quaker apostle dwelt mostly in a sphere apart, very little influenced by the thoughts, philosophical, poetical, or political, of the men of his stirring generation. The Bible seems to have been his only literature, and it may safely be said that Amos, the herdsman of Tekoa, who was separated from him by an interval of twenty-four centuries, had definitely more influence on his mind than William Shakespeare, who died but eight years before he came into the world.

' So too, for the political events of his time. . . . The Civil War began when Fox was in the eighteenth year of his age, and lasted till about the time when he began his missionary journeys. Yet to all these events he makes no allusion, and it may be doubted

---

[1] Robert Barclay, *op. cit.*, pp. 214, 215.

whether even at the time they greatly moved him.   The history
of his own soul, his struggles with the power of darkness, his
reachings forth after the light and peace of God, seem to have
absorbed all his thoughts, and the thunderstorms of war and
revolution crashed round him unheeded '.[1]

Probably the correct interpretation of the facts lies between
these extremes.   It is certainly impossible to believe that
a man with Fox's endowments and interests could have been
the detached individual of Hodgkin's picture ; only mental
deficiency or obsession could so remove a person from his
social environment, and there are certainly no evidences
of either in the case of Fox.   On the other hand, it is not
at all necessary to suppose that there was conscious borrowing ; the image, for instance, of the Flaming Sword, is
obviously inspired both in Boehme and in Fox by the
passage in Genesis iii. 24,[2] and it was almost certainly a
spontaneous emergence in both experiences of imagery
that was part of their mental equipment.   The important
point for the present purpose has been expressed by W. C.
Braithwaite in the following words :

' . . . No direct contact of Familist or Boehmist influences
with Fox has yet been established, nor would be likely to have
been alluded to in his *Journal*, had it occurred. He may most
probably have come into some knowledge of their ideas, but it is
important to bear in mind that these would be to him like other
" notions " until they became matters of heart-experience, and
when he had thus made them his own he would think no longer
of their human origin, and would speak of them as " openings "
of light to himself. . . . As Dr. R. M. Jones points out, any
knowledge of Boehme or of the Familist principles which came
to Fox through the small mystical sects and the current mystical
literature of the time might readily act on his spirit by way of
" suggestion " and be reproduced in a vivid psychic experience
which would be in his mind the sure evidence of its truth '.[3]

[1] Thomas Hodgkin, *op. cit.*, p. 16.
[2] In the Revised Version : ' . . . he placed at the east of the garden of
Eden the Cherubim, and the flame of a sword which turned every way,
to keep the way of the tree of life.'
[3] W. C. Braithwaite, *op. cit.*, p. 41, p. 42.

In other words, Fox was very definitely influenced by his environment, both religious and political. What was original in him was the selective interest and constructive imagination which dealt with the material of his environment in a particular and individual way. His religious experience was, beyond all question, original in the sense of first-hand—it was not a matter of conscious imitation and conformity. In the expression he gave to the felt realities of his experience, he was influenced, probably unconsciously, by the ideas of other individuals and groups. And more than this. What Freud has called the ' reality-principle ' was very marked in Fox, and what he was responding to in his religious behaviour was no mere subjective drama in his own soul—as Hodgkin seems to suggest—but the complex situation of the world of real men and women *as he perceived and imagined* that world. What characterizes and particularizes Fox is the fact, not that he ' dwelt mostly in a sphere apart, very little influenced by the thoughts, philosophical, poetical, or political, of the men of his stirring generation ', but that he saw more in the situation than most of his fellows. He was sensitive to precisely that ' beyond element ' in the situation which rendered all conventional and established responses to it unavailing and futile. The ordinary Puritan—whether Presbyterian, Anglican or Independent—and the ordinary Royalist—whether of the extreme or the moderate type— could react adequately along the lines of existing individual and group tendencies, and express themselves in controversy, conformity, conflict. To Fox, those elements in the situation which could be thus reacted to were almost entirely overshadowed by something more, and other, and this discrimination, as will be shewn in due course, produced in him in the first instance a marked affective state, with depression and anxiety, until later the ' beyond element ' was systematized by what is, in its psychological aspect, the work of fantasy, taking the form of imaginative insight and interpretation. The dominant element for Fox is, then, the relationship between man and the Power beyond which he now imaginatively discovers within as the Inner Light. In the process of this interpretation and discovery there are visions, voices, and other unusual phenomena which often characterize an intense experience of frustration superseded by religious construction, and which have already been noticed in the study of the Peyote Cult.

From this brief survey of the main features of the environment as it affected Fox, I now turn to the material incorporated in his *Journal*. There are many points in which the general trend of events within Fox's experience as here pourtrayed resembles that of John Rave and the Peyote eaters. The environment is a different and more intricate one ; the group tendencies which operated in Fox's *milieu* are more varied ; the situation to which he responded was mediated more through ideational than through purely perceptual channels, but in essence the psychological character of the experience and reaction is similar. Rave's instability (and sensitiveness) was noted and the suggestion was made that this was an indispensable individual characteristic in the initiator of a religious reconstruction or expansion. This character is even more marked in Fox, often approaching to abnormal intensity. While in the case of Rave the ' beyond element ' was almost thrust upon him by the objective nature of the peyote and its effects, in the case of Fox the discrimination is of a more vague and general character at first, and is accompanied by a more or less prolonged period of doubt, uncertainty and inquiry. But just as an integral part of Rave's experience was intense affect and suffering in the frustration of his normal powers of reaction, so it is with Fox. And in both cases the affect is followed by visions, and the final attainment of a state of bliss and perfect confidence. The parallel will become clear in tracing the course of events in Fox's experience as they bear upon, and express, his personal traits.

It is of considerable interest and importance, in view of current Psychoanalytical theories, to raise the question of sex instinct in connection with Fox. It has been easy to shew that thwarted, repressed and sublimated sex instinct has played a considerable part in determining the form of the religious experience of many persons, perhaps especially mystics,[1] but the conclusion that religion is always a form of substitute satisfaction for thwarted sex interest would require a great deal more evidence than yet has been offered. What seems to be established beyond question is the fact that the deprivation of normal satisfaction to the organism along any line of instinctive activity tends to promote an inner disturbance which, in the case of man, finds compensatory outlet in fantasy thinking. The importance of a deprivation of the nutritive instinct in fasting has already been displayed as a regular means of gaining religious experience, and asceticism in general has been a recognized means in all religions of securing special insight, knowledge, and experience of things beyond the normal. As the sex instinct is, in normal cases, one of the strongest, it is not wonderful that it tends to play an

[1] R. H. Thouless, *An Introduction to the Psychology of Religion*, 1923, chap. X. See also Footnote to p. 2 above. Also: C. G. Jung, *Analytical Psychology* (2nd ed. London, 1917), pp. 172-4, and 462-3.

important part in religious experience, just as it has been shewn by Freud to play an extremely important part in the psycho-neuroses. But that every kind of religious experience is determined by some irregular, repressed or sublimated sex interest is as great an exaggeration as the original Freudian theory that all psycho-neuroses are directly due to some disturbance in sexual function. On this matter Rivers wrote :

' The first result of the dispassionate study of the psycho-neuroses of warfare, in relation to Freud's scheme, was to show that in the vast majority of cases there is no reason to suppose that factors derived from the sexual life played any essential part in causation, but that these disorders became explicable as the result of the disturbance of another instinct, one even more fundamental than that of sex—the instinct of self-preservation, especially those forms of it which are adapted to protect the animal from danger. Warfare makes fierce onslaughts on an instinct or group of instincts which is rarely touched by the ordinary life of the member of a modern civilized community. War calls into activity processes and tendencies which in its absence would have lain wholly dormant '.[1]

I have been maintaining throughout this book that it is not the violent disturbance of instinctive function, in one or many directions, that characterizes religion, but the temporary frustration of all instincts and other active tendencies by the discrimination of something which is not specific enough to arouse any definite tendency, and which does not, therefore, involve the conflict between existing tendencies which is characteristic, for example, in the war situation. The typical nuclear religious experience is thus a kind of aching helplessness. The development, strength and inter-relation of the instincts and tendencies is obviously of importance in giving form and intensity to the frustration experience, but the conflict aroused by the

[1] *Instinct and the Unconscious*, pp. 4, 5.

stimulation simultaneously of rival instincts would never give rise to the fundamental experience of religion. In this matter George Fox affords a valuable instance of the inadequacy of the pan-sexual method of explanation, for all the evidence of the *Journal*, positive and negative, goes to shew that the psycho-sexual tendencies in him were, if not deficient, at least not strong enough to require any repression. He tells us of ' a gravity and stayedness of mind and spirit ' in his very young years ' not usual in children ', while

> ' When I came to eleven years of age, I knew pureness and righteousness ; for while a child I was taught how to walk to be kept pure '.[1]

This positive assertion gains in significance by the fact that there is nowhere any mention of concern about ' sin ' : as Dr. R. M. Jones says :

> ₁ It is surely a significant fact that, with all his sensitiveness of spirit, he never appears to have undergone any travail over his own sins, nor to have passed through that experience of conviction of sin which was such a common feature of the evangelical Christianity of his time '.[2]

It is significant, for it argues for a harmony of vital impulses which, judging from many other religious experiences, as well as from our knowledge of normal childhood, is at least unusual in so high a degree. All outer manifestations of sex interest and activity may be repressed—as indeed they usually are—but that is frequently, if not invariably, one of the conditions inducing a sense of guilt and a conviction of sin. In Fox's case there are no signs of any repression : by native endowment he was more active along the lines of other original tendencies.

---

[1] *The Journal of George Fox*, Tercentenary Text, edited by Norman Penney, 1924.
[2] *Beginnings of Quakerism*, Introd., p. xxxii.

' When I was come down into Leicestershire (he records) my relations would have had me marry, but I told them I was but a lad, and I must get wisdom '.[1]

There is no further indication of any interest directly or indirectly sexual till chapter xx, which begins :

' I had seen from the Lord a considerable time before that I should take Margaret Fell to be my wife '.[2]

But in this sex interest there is none of the passion of a strong instinct. His marriage relationship has all the characteristics of a mental and spiritual comradeship, accentuated and coloured, no doubt, by the facts of sex difference, but in all probability quite as much conditioned by gregariousness as sex. The fact is clear that once Fox's native tendencies were released by the attainment of the liberating experience of the reality and practical nature of religion, they functioned harmoniously and systematically, without any outstanding conflicts, repressions or sublimations. As Dr. Rachel Knight says :

' Fear became the essence of reverence for him. . . . Anger in Fox was as strong as in the most pugnacious of his fellow-men. But he had put such a curb of control upon it that, enraged at the incivility of a priest, he did not storm or fight, but was " wrapped up as in a rapture ". His refined instinct—torn asunder from coarser expressive reaction—could express itself in love even for personal persecutors. It could develop in him an attitude whereby he lived in the spirit that took away the occasion for all wars.

' George Fox's instinctive biological demands for food and drink blossomed out into a demand for spiritual rather than material values. You *can't kill an instinct*, and in him the physical thirst, which he refused to use in the conventional way for social drinking, became a double thirst. He thirsted for human companionship and for the presence of the Lord. . . .

' He was happy in the possession of property sufficient to enable him to live his life and be no burden upon friends or relatives. Therefore his acquisitions took the form of gathering into his Truth a large following in whom he rejoiced. Men, not things, were the objects which he garnered into his treasury '.[3]

[1] *Journal*, p. 1. [2] *Op. cit.*, p. 263.
[3] *The Founder of Quakerism*, pp. 232-3.

While in regard to his sexual life she says :

> ' The energy that might normally have gone into family re-
> lationships in his early manhood, nature used in aiding him to
> carry each of his characteristics to a higher level. They all became
> so closely co-ordinated that he pulled himself apart from the
> tension of his divided self and found himself so unified that he
> seemed another person '.[1]

What this means in more definite terms is that owing to
his psycho-physiological endowment, interest expressed
itself in Fox most naturally and intensely through other
reactive tendencies than that of sex, and no effort or
expenditure of energy was required to divert sex interest
into other channels. Indeed, from the evidence of the
Journal, it looks as if interest derived from more general
gregarious tendencies, such as what Dr. Knight calls the
' thirst for human companionship ', was needed to fortify
his sex impulse.

Another preliminary question in connection with Fox's
original psychical constitution is that of a native religious
interest or bent.[2] The first two pages of the *Journal* make
it very clear that hereditary disposition and early training
co-operated in directing Fox towards religion. His father
had ' a seed of God in him ' and was called by the neighbours
' Righteous Christer ', while his mother came ' of the stock
of the martyrs '. In very young years he displayed
' gravity and stayedness " and a dislike of wantonness, and
he could declare already that ' the Lord shewed ' him to
keep himself away from all the pollutions and infidelities
of the time. So obviously had the bent of his mind and
spirit become that

> ' Afterwards, as I grew up, my relations thought to make me
> a priest '.[3]

---

[1] *The Founder of Quakerism*, p. 231.   [2] See above, p. 95, pp. 104-5.
[3] *Journal*, pp. 1-2.

There can be little doubt that the nature of this original
bent, as in the cases of St. Teresa and John Rave, is largely
a matter of marked sensitiveness and mental plasticity.
This may be justly regarded as a bent towards religion
apart from the influence of specific religious instruction,
for it is the condition necessary for those finer and fuller
discriminations which lead to the ' beyond element ', even
in the absence of definite traditions and instruction. That
Fox was sensitive and plastic to the verge of instability is
abundantly shewn in the *Journal*.[1] Definite traces of a
hysterical strain are found in several instances. Among
the ' priests ' to whom he resorted for enlightenment was

> ' one Macham, a priest in high account. He would needs give
> me some physic, and I was to have been let blood ; but they
> could not get one drop of blood from me, either in arms or head '.[2]

while in connection with the well-known Lichfield exploit
he records that

> ' there seemed to me to be a channel of blood running down the
> streets and the market place appeared like a pool of blood '.[3]

An even more striking instance occurs after the death of
one Brown, ' who had great prophecies and sights of me
upon his death-bed ',

> ' When this man was buried, a great work of the Lord fell upon
> me, to the admiration of many who thought I had been dead ;
> and many came to see me for about fourteen days' time. I was
> very much altered in countenance and person, as if my body had
> been new-moulded or changed '.[4]

A similar experience befell him later at Reading ;[5] and at
Mansfield he had a temporary hysterical blindness.[6]

The more important aspect of Fox's constitution, however, for my purpose, is his extreme sensitiveness, and it

---

[1] The evidence is summarized by R. M. Jones in Introd. to *The Beginnings
of Quakerism*, pp. xxviii.–xxxi.   [2] *Journal*, p. 5.   [3] *Op. cit.*, p. 40.
[4] *Op. cit.*, p. 12.   [5] *Op. cit.*, p. 176.   [6] *Op. cit.*, p. 16.

is this which must be accepted as the entirely original or native element in Fox's religious bent. R. M. Jones says :

> ' The influence of heredity is no doubt a powerful factor, but a very large part of the mental equipment, once attributed to inheritance, is more properly assigned to these profoundly shaping processes, suggestion and imitation, through which the new-born individual takes to himself the ideas, activities, manners, customs, emotional traits, strivings, and *spirit* of the group which most impresses his life. . . .
> ' This is peculiarly the case with the type of persons who belong to the class of geniuses or creative leaders. They are always persons who are acutely sensitive to the spirit of their time, the subtle currents and inward strivings of their period. They are as responsive to group-tendencies as a sounding-box or a musical instrument to vibrations ; they are *suggestible* to a degree that ordinary thick-skinned mortals have no notion of '.[1]

But the point I would stress is that though the environment is ' no doubt a powerful factor ', it is quite incapable of inducing a religious response, or ' calling forth ' the character of creative leadership unless it bears upon a personality peculiarly endowed with a sensitiveness which is beyond the ordinary. That characteristic is at present not reducible to terms of simpler analysis, and must be accepted as fundamental.[2] Undoubtedly this is one of the more important sources of Fox's religious experience and response, as Dr. Rachel Knight has insisted in her chapter on ' Hypersensitivity of the Special Senses '. After citing evidence from the *Journal* she says :

> ' His senses were perhaps no more innately sensitive than those of ordinary men. But bombarded on all sides by insistent stimuli he had learned the use of them so that his sensory reach was more extensive and accurate than theirs '.[3]

And concludes :

> ' His God is not the transcendental God of Plotinus, however, whom he reaches out to touch with some special organ or sense.

[1] *Beginnings of Quakerism*, Introd., pp. xxvi.–vii.
[2] See Note added at end of Chapter, p. 166.
[3] *Founder of Quakerism*, p. 46-7.

He is immanent in the world and in his own life. Fox's life, it seems to me, is in full accordance with Locke's dictum that there is nothing in the life that is not in the senses. The rich soul life of Fox is but the refined behaviour of the special senses. Even the mystic seems to be usually aware of the truth of this '[1]

Nevertheless I differ from Dr. Knight on a point of psychological importance. She seems to treat sensitiveness as being in the main a matter of sensory acuity. She is probably right in stating that in this respect there can be an increase through learning, and therefore this characteristic is an acquired rather than an original one. But the sensitiveness which Fox, in common with other creative personalities, displays, is not a matter of the physiological efficiency of the senses, but a psychical sensitiveness which makes possible the assimilation, retention, and organization of material, however communicated or derived, in a fuller and deeper measure than is usual, and which no amount of practice can bring about. This is no doubt connected with the arrangement, inter-relationship and integration of the inherited psychical dispositions, and it becomes possible for the person so endowed to discriminate more than is ever sensed : a capacity developed to some extent in everyone, for without it perception would be impossible, but which reaches a maximum degree in relatively few. Most poets, for example, are probably characterized by a heightened sensory acuity, which gives them their joy in nature, and their ability to describe and celebrate it in a fashion beyond the capacity of less sensitive persons precisely because they actually see, hear, and smell more than others do. But this does not necessarily reach the intensity of that sensitiveness which characterizes the religious seer, in which there is an awareness or discrimin-

[1] *Founder of Quakerism*, pp. 55–6.

ation of the fact, first *felt*, and only in any way cognized after fantasy and imagination have supervened, that there is more in or behind nature than is within the scope either of the senses to receive or the existing tendencies to react to. The poetry of Sir Walter Scott—and the prose as well —is characterized by vivid descriptions of nature, but there is no indication of the mystic's vision beyond transforming the poet's description into the language of religion, as is the case with Wordsworth, for example. The contrast may be illustrated by brief quotations of typical passages from each.

> ' The western waves of ebbing day
> Rolled o'er the glen their level way ;
> Each purple peak, each flinty spire,
> Was bathed in floods of living fire.
> But not a setting beam could glow
> Within the dark ravines below,
> Where twined the path in shadow hid,
> Round many a rocky pyramid,
> Shooting abruptly from the dell
> Its thunder-splintered pinnacle ;
> Round many an insulated mass,
> The native bulwarks of the pass,
> Huge as the tower which builders vain
> Presumptuous piled on Shinar's plain.
> The rocky summits, split and rent,
> Formed turret, dome, or battlement ;
> Or seemed fantastically set
> With cupola or minaret,
> Wild crests as pagod ever decked,
> Or mosque of Eastern architect '.[1]

Here Scott's vivid appreciation of the beauty and interest of nature is apparent, and every indication that he sees more of nature than an average observer ; but his imagery is derived from the realm of human activity and art ; it is saturated in Scott's dominant interest in the history of

[1] *The Lady of the Lake*, Canto I., xi.

chivalry and war ; it never takes the imagination out into the infinite.

> ' For I have learn'd
> To look on Nature, not as in the hour
> Of thoughtless youth ; but hearing oftentimes
> The still, sad music of humanity,
> Not harsh nor grating, though of ample power
> To chasten and subdue. And I have felt
> A presence that disturbs me with the joy
> Of elevated thoughts ; a sense sublime
> Of something far more deeply interfused,
> Whose dwelling is the light of setting suns,
> And the round ocean, and the living air,
> And the blue sky, and in the mind of man :
> A motion and a spirit, that impels
> All thinking things, all objects of all thought,
> And rolls through all things '.[1]

This is not description of nature, but the record of a vision which sees beyond the appearances, however lovely, of nature, and communicates the living thrill of the experience in the language of mysticism. Nor is it solely mystical language. In the lines ' I have felt A presence that disturbs me with the joy Of elevated thoughts ', we have a psychologically exact account of the experience of that ' beyond element ' in the situation which has been so much stressed in these pages. It is at first simply *feeling*, most truly described as ' *disturbance* ' until there comes the play of imagery and thought about the feeling, which builds it up into ' a sense sublime Of something far more deeply interfused, Whose dwelling is the light of setting suns '. Here is a sensitiveness which is other than a mere sensory acuity : it is a power of intuition, in Lévy-Bruhl's expression, which gives ' implicit faith in *the presence and agency* of powers which are invisible and inaccessible to the senses '.[2]

---

[1] *Lines Composed a Few Miles Above Tintern Abbey.*

[2] See Footnote to page 80 above. *Cf.* also W. R. Inge, *The Psychology of Faith*, p. 53 : ' Faith, then, " transcends experience " ; it appears as a constructive activity. It employs the imagination to fill out what is wanting in experience.'

Now it is precisely this type of discrimination, or intuition, which characterizes Fox as he reveals himself and his experience in the *Journal*: it is this which places him apart from the skilful observer (who may be his equal in sensory power) and the critic, and puts him in the rank of the constructive and original seers. And for the purpose of the present investigation this is the crucial matter. Others have utilized the material of Fox's *Journal* for general biographical purposes (as, for instance, Hodgkin and Braithwaite), and for a general psychological investigation (as, for instance, Dr. Rachel Knight), but so far as I am aware it has not been utilized to display the operation of a native ability for the kind of discrimination or intuition I have postulated, which involves, and indeed is part of, the experience of frustration at the hands of a universe which is, as it were, challenging man with signals for responding to which he has no finished native disposition or tendency, but the experience of which implies a first step in the process of devising a new response and achieving an expanded consciousness.

The first few pages of the *Journal* are, from this point of view, remarkable. Already in his ' very young years ' Fox was precocious enough to observe a lightness and wantonness among old men which hardly occurs to the ordinary child. But more than this, he discriminates in this situation something which induces in him a powerful enough affective reaction to make him determine

' If ever I come to be a man, surely I shall not do so, nor be so wanton '.[1]

By the time he was eleven years of age this affective reaction to the moral situation has already been interpreted

[1] *Journal*, p. 1.

in the more or less conventional forms of current religious teaching. He is able to say :

> ‘ The Lord taught me to be faithful in all things, and to act faithfully two ways, viz., inwardly to God, and outwardly to man ; and to keep to Yea and Nay in all things. For the Lord shewed me, that though the people of the world have mouths full of deceit, and changeable words, yet I was to keep to Yea and Nay in all things ; and that my words should be few and savoury, seasoned with grace ; and that I might not eat and drink to make myself wanton, but for health, using the creatures in their service as servants in their places, to the glory of Him that created them ; they being in their covenant, and I being brought up into the covenant, as sanctified by the Word which was in the beginning, by which all things are upheld ; wherein is unity with all creation ’.[1]

But it was when Fox was nineteen that he underwent a peculiarly intense affective experience in connection with a drinking party. His cousin and another ‘ professor’ [2] invited him to drink a jug of beer with them, and Fox, being of a sociable disposition, willingly complied. But

> ‘ When we had drunk a glass apiece they began to drink healths, calling for more, and agreeing together that he that would not drink should pay all. I was grieved that any who made profession of religion should do so. They grieved me very much, having never had such a thing put to me before, by any sort of people ; wherefore I rose up to be gone, and putting my hand into my pocket, laid a groat on the table before them, and said : “ If it be so, I’ll leave you ”. So I went away ; and when I had done what business I had to do, I returned home, but did not go to bed that night, nor could not sleep, but sometimes walked up and down, and sometimes prayed and cried to the Lord, who said unto me : “ Thou seest how young people go together unto vanity, and old people into the earth ; thou must forsake all, both young and old, and keep out of all, and be as a stranger unto all ” ’.[3]

Now, as ordinarily apprehended by an ordinary person, there is nothing in this situation to produce so profound an upheaval. Its effect on Fox was clearly due to the fact that it stood for far more to him than it would have done to another. And it not merely stood for something which

---

[1] *Journal*, pp. 1–2.
[2] The term Fox uses for one who professes Christianity.
[3] *Op. cit.*, p. 2–3.

he could object to, protest against, and so dispose of. The something which created in him this profound disturbance overwhelmed him with its vast though vague significance. The drinking bout was a sign of the times : an instance of the fact that the people around him ' did not possess what they professed '. If Fox had no sort of consciousness of personal sin, he early awakened to a consciousness of evil in the world which weighed on his spirit to an extraordinary degree, and he felt that evil in relation to something outside the realm of mere human misdoing, as this excessive reaction to the drinking bout shews. A less sensitive person, however his early training and moral interests might lead him to react with disapproval and even disgust to this situation, would not experience so profound an upheaval as to cause a sleepless night and an experience of agonizing before God. He would respond to the situation with some more or less drastic act of protest and disapproval, and in that response dispose of the matter. The features of the situation which Fox discriminated admitted of no such conclusive response. True he left the party, and thereby indicated his disapproval ; but that was a response only to the most superficial aspect as it affected Fox. It seems to me that we have here clear evidence that Fox was, probably unconsciously, affected to the depths of his being by the larger situation in England as a whole, and this incident acted as an occasion for that unconsciously incubating discrimination to manifest itself in the form of intense emotional disturbance. The times, as we have seen, were out of joint. The civil war was in process—confusion and conflict, suffering and distress, were rife. To an ordinarily sensitive person, capable of an average appreciation of the situation, the way was fairly clear for the application of such principles, or tendencies to respond, as had become established in the form of guiding sentiments. He would throw in his lot with one or other of the contending parties, and thus face the problems as he discriminated them along the lines of established reaction patterns. It is interesting to note that at the time when his parents would have had him marry,

> ' Others would have had me into the Auxiliary Band among the soldiery, but I refused ; and I was grieved that they proffered such things to me, being a tender youth '.[1]

But this appeal to Fox to respond to the needs of the times along the lines of the instinct of pugnacity was beside the mark, for the simple reason that what most affected him in the situation was something which baffled all his instincts and hitherto acquired tendencies. In other words, the situation which summoned the active participation of so many of the best people of the time in a war for liberty, or loyalty, as they may have seen it, simply brought about in Fox a condition of frustration. Thus

> ' . . . a strong temptation to despair came upon me. . . . But temptations grew more and more, and I was tempted almost to despair ; and when Satan could not effect his design upon me that way, he laid snares for me and baits to draw me to commit some sin, whereby he might take advantage to bring me to despair. I was about twenty years of age when these exercises came upon me ; and I continued in that condition some years, in great troubles, and fain I would have put it from me. I went to many a priest to look for comfort, but found no comfort from them '.[2]

In the course of his wanderings he came to London

> ' and was under great misery and trouble there ; for I looked upon the great professors of the city of London, and I saw all was dark and under the chain of darkness '.[3]

This state of depression and anxiety lasted for some time—some years in his own words. He visited his home, only

---

[1] *Journal*, p. 4.　　[2] *Op. cit.*, p. 3.　　[3] *Op. cit.*, p. 3.

to leave again for Coventry after the advice to marry, and to join the army. But

> ' After some time I went into my own country again, and was there about a year, in great sorrows and troubles, and walked many nights by myself '.[1]

The story of his eager quest among the ' priests ' for help and guidance shews his state of mind. What he wanted was to gain an experimental or first-hand knowledge which would dissipate the affect of frustration and release his personality for systematic action, and at first he hoped to find someone who, having shared his frustration experience, could ' speak to his condition '. But the priests completely failed to meet his need. The ' ancient priest at Mancetter ' who bade him ' take tobacco and sing psalms ' evidently thought his difficulties were indications of mental aberration, while the priest Macham, already referred to, clearly diagnosed a state of derangement. Fox's state of mind was uncomprehended by these folk precisely because they did not share his deeper discrimination of the times. To them it was a conflict in politics and a struggle of rival religious forms. To Fox it was something which was literally *unutterably* more.

After his disappointment with the priests we hear of the first ' openings ' :

> ' About the beginning of the year 1646, as I was going to Coventry and entering towards the gate, a consideration arose in me, how it was said that all Christians are believers, both Protestants and Papists ; and the Lord opened to me that, if all were believers, then they were all born of God, and passed from death to life, and that none were true believers but such ; and though others said they were believers, yet they were not. At another time, as I was walking in a field on a First-day morning, the Lord opened to me that being bred at Oxford or Cambridge was not enough to fit and qualify men to be ministers of Christ ; and

[1] *Op. cit.*, p. 4.

I stranged at it, because it was the common belief of people. But I saw it clearly as the Lord opened it to me, and was satisfied, and admired the goodness of the Lord who had opened this thing unto me that morning.   This struck at priest Stephens' ministry.'[1]

This marks a very interesting and important stage in Fox's experience. It shews him at the point of breaking loose from his childhood's attitude towards the authority of traditional teaching. Already, it is true, that breaking loose had begun when he left home and kindred to wander on his pilgrimage, but the whole attitude of his mind was still one of dependence upon outward authority. He hoped and expected to be able to get instruction which would give him understanding of that which had so deeply affected him, but which still remained a vaguely felt disturbance of the whole mental life rather than a recognizable problem to face and solve. But his experience with his own priest Stephens, who

' would applaud and speak highly of me to others ; and what I said in discourse to him on the week-days he would preach of on the First-days ; for which I did not like him ',[2]

brought him to the realization that the preaching of this priest was the outcome of nothing more authoritative than the thoughts and considerations which welled up in his own mind. It is a significant experience, and one by no means uncommon with young people brought up in a religious environment. From the general tone and atmosphere they are led to suppose that there is some very peculiar and special character attaching to ' professors ', and still more to ministers of religion, and the discovery, when it comes, that the minds of such people work in the same way as their own, and that preaching is often simply the expression of opinions received from others, or fabricated and built

[1] *Journal*, pp. 5–6.   [2] *Journal*, p. 4.

up in the mind by ordinary processes of thought, is apt to have far-reaching effects. It may lead either to a rejection of the whole edifice of religion, or to a completely new view of its nature and the mode of its experience. What seems to have happened in Fox's case is that the discovery completely destroyed his faith in 'priests' and 'professors' as such, but left him in a condition of heightened receptivity to the influences of thought welling up in himself, provided he did not consciously fabricate them. He was no more prepared to trust his own intellectual gropings than he was those of others : it was the felt inadequacy of his own efforts which destroyed his confidence in the priests when he discovered that it was on such material as this that they depended. Here, then, we find Fox very much in the condition of the Seekers—detached from all forms and external authorities, yet expecting that somehow the supreme reality would make itself known, and not remain a mere vaguely felt somewhat. And the awareness of this general fact itself came to Fox, not as the result of consciously thinking out the issues. The recognition that true belief was not a matter of guaranteed opinions, Protestant or Papist, but was a matter of a definite divine operation, emerged into his consciousness, as it were, ready-made. The thought, or consideration, had its psychic connections with Fox's mental life as a whole, but the premises were unconsciously elaborated, until some particular experience opened the way for the conclusion to appear in consciousness. In that sense, Fox's term, 'opening', is peculiarly appropriate. And since there was no obvious context of mental effort involved in achieving the result, Fox at once accepted the thought as a communication from the Beyond, and an opening from the Lord.

The second opening, concerning qualifications for the ministry of Christ, displays even more clearly all these features. Fox did not consciously realize that his experience with the priests had destroyed his whole attitude of confidence in theological education and ordination—but that in fact was what had happened. Probably Priest Stephens did more than any other single person to initiate in Fox the process of unconscious mentation whose end-result burst into consciousness as the conclusion about the ministry and its qualifications. But the conclusion was so completely dissociated from all conscious context as well as from prevailing popular opinion, that Fox ' stranged ' at it. And the important thing is that this sort of invasion of consciousness was accepted by Fox as the mode in which God communicated with men ; hence we find that after these preliminary ' openings ' there follow many more. Fox, that is, expects and relies on, such up-surgings from the unconscious. The matter of these openings may have had their importance—and doubtless did—but much more fundamental for Fox's after experience was their mode. As in the philosophy of Descartes, the *cogito ergo sum* is not of primary importance as an argument in favour of the existence of a thinking, or conscious being, but because it provides the type of intuitive certitude which can become the test of truth,[1] so the conviction that true believers must be ' born of God ', and true ministers have something other than an Oxford or Cambridge education was chiefly of importance in that the mode in

[1] Robert Adamson, in *The Development of Modern Philosophy*, 1908, in discussing the *cogito ergo sum* formula, says : ' Wherever we find, then, in understanding, in what is intuitively apprehended, as clear and inevitable and indubitable a connexion as is contained in the fundamental datum, we shall accept it as so far an indication of truth, and of truth respecting real existence ' (p. 12).

which they were communicated to consciousness provided the criterion of a divine revelation or utterance.

But the way was by no means clear yet. The unconscious, which is the workshop in which the raw material of experience is fabricated into many forms, does not only yield to consciousness completed thoughts or images which can vindicate themselves as ' openings ' from God. There were further discriminations for Fox to make before he could arrive at his formulation of the Inner Light. He experienced uprushes of quite another character. Very significant is his reference to the people

' that relied much on dreams. I told them, except they could distinguish between dream and dream, they would mash or confound all together ; for there were three sorts of dreams : multitude of business sometimes caused dreams ; and there were whisperings of Satan in man in the night-seasons ; and there were speakings of God to man in dreams ',[1]

especially in connection with the fact which he goes on many times to record, that

' though I had great openings, yet great trouble and temptation came many times upon me, so that when it was day I wished for night, and when it was night I wished for day. . . .

' But my troubles continued, and I was often under great temptations ; I fasted much, and walked abroad in solitary places many days, and often took my Bible, and went and sate in hollow trees and lonesome places till night came on ; and frequently, in the night, walked mournfully about by myself : for I was a man of sorrows in the times of the first workings of the Lord in me.

' Though my exercises and troubles were very great, yet they were not so continual but that I had some intermissions, and was sometimes brought into such a heavenly joy, that I thought I had been in Abraham's bosom. As I cannot declare the misery I was in, it was so great and heavy upon me, so neither can I set forth the mercies of God unto me in all my misery '.[2]

Hitherto the process had been very largely a negative one. The experience of profound disturbance resulting from the

[1] *Journal*, p. 7.   [2] *Op. cit.*, pp. 7 and 8.

discrimination of elements in the total situation which were ' beyond ' the range of predispositions for response remains, though the first indications have come that the grasp upon that reality beyond must be a matter of first-hand personal experience. The consciousness of this fact, indeed, came in so urgent a form, dissociated so entirely from all conscious context, that it was itself treated as an ' opening ' from God. But there was as yet no sufficient interpretation of the mysterious and beyond element to organize Fox's practical tendencies for systematic response. He was still in the condition of frustration, involving partially suspended (or undirected) activity. He may at times have rejoiced in some uprush into consciousness of a truth, an image, an idea, a faith, that for its beauty and unexpectedness had all the marks of an opening ; but he was none the less withheld and thwarted by frequent experiences of the emergence into consciousness of other kinds of idea— temptations to despair, feelings of sorrow, misery, and the like. The great act of imaginative insight and construction which brought the Beyond into the range of practical and continuous response by all the faculties of his personality— the vision, imagination, idea, or conviction that the Light of God was within, and that it could illuminate all that was strange and mysterious without, and that Christ Himself speaks and teaches within the soul—was still delayed.

It is of extreme interest and importance to note that while Fox was beginning to experience the uprushes from the unconscious which he calls ' openings ', and yet was still suffering from ' great troubles and temptations ', he adopted, apparently without any conscious recognition of its technical significance, the age-old method of fasting.

Having travelled into Nottinghamshire, he records that :

' I met with a tender people, and a very tender woman, whose name was Elizabeth Hooton ; and with these I had some meetings and discourses. But my troubles continued, and I was often under great temptations ; I fasted much. . . .'[1]

It is surely significant that very soon after this account of recourse to fasting the crucial experience comes to Fox. His faith destroyed in the priests, he turned to the Dissenting people, but soon he left the Separate preachers also,

' for I saw that there was none among them all that could speak to my condition '.[2]

The *Journal* proceeds :

' And when all my hopes in them and in all men were gone, so that I had nothing outwardly to help me, nor could I tell what to do ; then, oh ! then I heard a voice which said : " There is one, even Christ Jesus, that can speak to thy condition : " and when I heard it, my heart did leap for joy. Then the Lord did let me see why there was none upon the earth that could speak to my condition, namely, that I might give Him all the glory ; for all are concluded under sin, and shut up in unbelief, as I had been, that Jesus Christ might have the pre-eminence, who enlightens, and gives grace and faith and power. Thus when God doth work, who shall let it ? and this I knew experimentally. My desires after the Lord grew stronger, and zeal in the pure knowledge of God, and of Christ alone, without the help of any man, book, or writing. For though I read the scriptures that spake of Christ and of God, yet I knew Him not, but by revelation, as He who hath the key did open, and as the Father of Life drew me to His Son by His Spirit. Then the Lord gently led me along, and let me see His love, which was endless and eternal, surpassing all the knowledge that men have in the natural state, or can get by history or books ; and that love let me see myself, as I was without Him. I was afraid of all company, for I saw them perfectly where they were, through the love of God, which let me see myself '.[3]

This is a culminating point in Fox's experience. We have passed the stage of the openings, and now enter that of the visions—though this first of the new experiences is not in the form of a hallucinated vision, but of a hallucinated

[1] *Journal*, p. 7.　　[2] *Op. cit.*, p. 8.　　[3] *Op. cit.*, p. 8.

voice. There is no reason to suppose that Fox is here
speaking metaphorically. If the hearing of the voice meant
simply an uprush from the unconscious of the same kind
as the conviction about believers and priests, there is no
reason to doubt that Fox would have introduced this as
another opening from the Lord. But as he definitely
claims to have heard a voice speaking to him, and as it
caused his heart to ' leap for joy ', we may take it that he
did hear the voice : or, in the terms of a purely empirical
psychology, that he suffered an auditory hallucination.
That is to say, on this occasion, there was an objective
projection of an unconsciously elaborated conclusion in a
form which had the value of an auditory perception.
Physiologically, what may be supposed to have taken place
is a centrally initiated stimulation of the auditory centres
of the brain. But, in fact, we have to deal with something
which is much more complicated than a physiological
curiosity or a psychological hallucination, namely a psychical event which was a transforming experience for Fox as
a person. Never again did he have in the same way the
experience of complete frustration. It is true that in his
next recorded vision of the ' great love of God ' he was at
one time tempted again to despair, and was ' in great
perplexity and trouble for many days ', but with this difference from the earlier period of prolonged depression—' yet
I gave myself to the Lord still '. Moreover, he goes on :

' One day when I had been walking solitarily abroad, and was
come home, I was taken up in the love of God, so that I could
not but admire the greatness of His love. While I was in that
condition it was opened unto me by the eternal light and power,
and I saw clearly therein that all was done, and to be done, in
and by Christ ; and how He conquers and destroys this tempter,
the Devil, and all his works, and is atop of him ; and that all
these troubles were good for me, and temptation for the trial of
my faith, which Christ had given me. When at any time my

condition was veiled, my secret belief was stayed firm, and hope underneath held me as an anchor in the bottom of the sea, and anchored my immortal soul to its Bishop, causing it to swim above the sea, the world, where all the raging waves, foul weather, tempests, and temptations are. But, oh! then did I see my troubles, trials and temptations more than ever I had done. As the light appeared, all appeared that is out of the light; darkness, death, temptations, the unrighteous, the ungodly; all was manifest and seen in the light. Then after this, there did a pure fire appear in me : then I saw how He sate as a refiner's fire and as fuller's soap ; then the spiritual discerning came into me, by which I did discern my own thoughts, groans and sighs ; and what it was that did veil me, and what it was that did open me. That which could not abide in the patience nor endure the fire, in the light I found to be the groans of the flesh that could not give up to the will of God, which had veiled me ; and that could not be patient in all trials, troubles and anguishes and perplexities, and could not give up self to die by the cross, the power of God, that the living and quickened might follow Him ; and that which would cloud and veil from the presence of Christ—that which the sword of the Spirit cuts down, and which must die—might not be kept alive '.[1]

The importance of fasting in connection with the induction of fantasy and hallucination has already been noted in reference to the Winnebago fasting practices. It is clear here also that there is a definite connection between Fox's hallucination and his fasting. Can any account of this connection be given ? It has been shewn that he was in a state of depression and anxiety, as a result of the more or less continuous experience of frustration. But in the meanwhile he did not reach a condition of complete collapse, which would be the ultimate goal of absolute frustration, and this means that in spite of much unconscious effort to grapple with the ' beyond ' elements (effort which manifested itself in consciousness as the affect, depression, anxiety, etc.) there was still a certain amount of normal activity going on ; that is, Fox was carrying out adequate responses to the immediate, if

[1] *Journal*, pp. 9, 10.

minor, situations of life. Any further withdrawal of
interest from the ordinary features of the everyday situation would mean an accession of strength to the processes
of the unconscious, and a deprivation of the necessary
sustenance for renewing the energies of the organism
would also involve a weakening of the barriers between
conscious and unconscious ; it would promote a condition
in many ways resembling sleep, when the ordinary conscious standards of reality are in abeyance. In this condition, as we all know from experience, unconscious thought
discharges itself, as it were, into consciousness in intensely
dramatic form. It is here no matter of sudden ' inspira-
tions ', but of definite hallucinations. In precisely this
fashion Fox, as a result of fasting at such a juncture,
passed from the phase of the uprushes of *thought in the
form of ideas,* to that of the uprushes of *thought in the form
of voices heard and visions seen.* It is quite probable that
Fox made a practice of fasting, for he speaks of it as if
it were a regular part of his discipline[1]. And it is certain
that once initiated, this habit of hallucinating the products
of unconscious mentation continued with Fox. Instances
abound throughout the *Journal,* of which one may suffice
by way of illustration. Fox claims to have had a special
knowledge of the Restoration, not in the form of special
information, but in the form of a ' sight and sense '—
and this some time before the actual event. His words
are :

> ' I had a sight and sense of the King's return a good while
> before, and so had some others. . . . When several rash spirits
> that came amongst us would have bought Somerset House, that

---

[1] e.g. at Lancaster, in 1652 : ' At this time I was in a fast, and was
not to eat until this work of God, which then lay weighty upon me, was
accomplished.' *Journal,* p. 79.

we might have meetings in it, I forbade them to do so ; for I then foresaw the King's coming in again '.[1]

The ' sight and sense ' obviously were projected images of the return of the King ; where and how did these images originate in the first instance ? We have independent evidence which gives us very definitely the answer to this question. Ideas of the King's return had been received by Fox from the common expectation and expressed desires of multitudes of persons, and these ideas had been unconsciously elaborated by him. J. R. Green records that after the dissolution of the Parliament of 1654 there was real danger of a Royalist revolt :

' That a danger of Royalist revolt existed was undeniable, but the danger was at once doubled by the general discontent. From this moment, Whitelock tells us, " many sober and noble patriots ", in despair of public liberty, " did begin to incline to the King's restoration ". In the mass of the population the reaction was far more rapid. " Charles Stuart ", writes a Cheshire correspondent to the Secretary of State, " hath five hundred friends in these adjacent counties for every one friend to you among them " '.[2]

Fox did not consciously accept the notion as probable from his reading of the times and his intercourse with people, but he unconsciously assimilated the general expectation and wish, and then consciously became aware of his ' sight and sense ' of the King's return.

It seems, then, that the thing that resolved the situation for Fox, and brought him a certitude which nothing afterwards shook, was hallucinatory experience of a kind which released his personal activities and organized his tendencies around a practical objective. The evils and sufferings of the time which had weighed so heavily on

[1] *Op. cit.*, p. 175. Other instances of experiences more intense than ' openings,' illusions, premonitions and hallucinations are given on the following pages of the *Journal* : 9, 10, 11, 12, 13, 37, 39, 40, 57, 130, 153, 173, 176, 178, 196, 216, 235, 258, 260, 316.

[2] J. R. Green, *op. cit.*, p. 571.

his spirit—and which continued even to do so even after the transforming experience—were now brought within the range of active response by reason of a systematic interpretation, achieved through unconscious processes of assimilation and elaboration, and irradiating consciousness in the form of openings, and those more intense experiences of visions, voices and the like.   In the light of his ' openings ', and now still more of his intenser ' revelations ', it became clear to Fox that the distressing and hitherto uncomprehended situation was the outcome of the fact that

> ' many talked of the law who had never known the law to be their schoolmaster ; and many talked of the gospel of Christ who had never known life and immortality brought to light in them by it '.[1]

And the adequate and conclusive response to that situation, in the production of which Fox discerned a disharmony between human deed and divine intention, was to travel about and declare truth.   And this we find follows in the *Journal* :

> ' Passing on, I went among the professors at Dukinfield and Manchester, where I stayed a while, and declared Truth among them '.[2]

Still subject to temptations and sufferings, Fox records :

> ' I could find none to open my condition to but the Lord alone, unto Whom I cried night and day.   I went back into Nottinghamshire, and there the Lord shewed me that the natures of those things which were hurtful without, were within, in the hearts and minds of wicked men.   I cried to the Lord, saying : " Why should I be thus, seeing I was never addicted to commit those evils ? " and the Lord answered that it was needful I should have a sense of all conditions, and in this I saw the infinite love of God '.[3]

Yet he was now actively engaged in ' declaring truth,' for people came

---

[1] *Journal*, p. 10.   [2] *Op. cit.*, p. 11.   [3] *Op. cit.*, p. 11.

' from far and near to see me ; but I was fearful of being drawn out by them ; yet I was made to speak and open things to them '.[1]

It was at this time that the prolonged strain of his experience culminated in the seizure after the prophecies of Brown on his death-bed. Here again the abnormal psychological condition was one which did not lead Fox to a ' flight from reality ', but one which gave him further imaginative insight into reality of such a kind as to facilitate his work :

> ' While I was in that condition, I had a sense and discerning given me by the Lord, through which I saw plainly, that when many people talked of God and Christ, etc., the serpent spake in them ; but this was hard to be borne '.[2]

This is an interesting instance in which a previous ' opening ' concerning the real ignorance of many who spoke of the law, and the gospel of Christ (see last page) recurs during a period of special sensitiveness in an intensified form, bringing with it a definite affect of resentment which added force to Fox's counter proclamation of ' Truth '. Thus :

> ' . . . the work of the Lord went on in some, and my sorrows and troubles began to wear off, and tears of joy dropped from me, so that I could have wept night and day with tears of joy to the Lord, in humility and brokenness of heart. I saw into that which was without end, and things which cannot be uttered, and of the greatness and infiniteness of the love of God, which cannot be exprest by words. For I had been brought through the very ocean of darkness and death, and through and over the power of Satan, by the eternal, glorious power of Christ ; even through that darkness was I brought, which covered-over all the world, and which chained down all, and shut up all in the death. The same eternal power of God, which brought me through these things, was that which afterwards shook the nations, priests, professors, and people '.[3]

This very clearly indicates the truth of the thesis that in proportion as the diffused affective state of frustration,

---

[1] *Op. cit.*, p. 12.　　[2] *Op. cit.*, p. 12.　　[3] *Op. cit.*, p. 12.

with its occasional openings, yielded to a condition of
fresh practical adaptation to the situation through imaginative formulation, accompanied by specific affect, and Fox
was able to respond actively to what he now could recognize
as the fundamental meaning of the situation, the anxiety
and depression gave place to confidence and faith and a
state of bliss.   He can now find abundant outlet for his
interest because he has at length brought the strange,
baffling and mysterious elements of the situation within
the scope of his practical tendencies.   When on one
occasion he is thwarted in his intended action at Mansfield,
where

> ' it was upon me from the Lord to go and speak to the justices,
> that they should not oppress the servants in their wages ',[1]

it so deeply affected him that he was smitten with hysterical blindness.   Indeed, what now supervenes is a difficulty
in selecting the mode of response to the challenge of the
times and its needs, for after the experience quoted in the
comparison with Boehme (pages 128-9) he says :

> ' I was at a stand in my mind whether I should practise physic
> for the good of mankind, seeing the nature and virtues of the
> creatures were so opened to me by the Lord '.[2]

[1] *Op. cit.*, p. 16.

[2] *Op. cit.*, p. 17.   An interesting parallel to this case of indetermination
after a great enlightenment is afforded in the story of Gotama.   After
the Great Enlightenment beneath the Bo Tree, the Buddha is reported
to have hesitated whether to attempt to proclaim the way of release
which had revealed itself to him, since it is ' profound, recondite, and
difficult of comprehension. . . . Mankind, on the other hand, is captivated,
entranced, held spell-bound by its lusts,' and therefore ' it is hard for them
to understand the law of dependence on assignable reasons, the doctrine
of Dependent Origination,' etc.   ' If I were to teach the Doctrine, others
would fail to understand me, and my vexation and trouble would be
great.'
   ' Thus, O priests, did I ponder, and my mind was disinclined to action,
and to any proclaiming of the Doctrine.
   ' Then, O priests, Brahma Sahampati perceived what was in my mind,
and it occurred to him as follows :
   ' " Lo, the world is lost, is ruined !   For the mind of The Tathagata,

This practical difficulty received its solution in the course of a short time, and through the process of unconscious elaboration :

'While I was there (in Leicestershire, in the vale of Beavor) the Lord opened to me three things, relating to those three great professions in the world—physic, divinity (so called), and law. He shewed me that the physicians were out of the wisdom of God, by which the creatures were made ; and so knew not their virtues, because they were out of the word of wisdom, by which they were made. He shewed me that the priests were out of the true faith, which Christ is the author of ; the faith which purifies and gives victory, and brings people to have access to God, by which they please God ; which mystery of faith is held in a pure conscience. He shewed me also, that the lawyers were out of the equity, and out of the true justice, and out of the law of God, which went over the first transgression, and over all sin, and answered the Spirit of God, that was grieved and transgressed in man. And that these three, the physicians, the priests and the lawyers, ruled the world out of the wisdom, out of the faith, and out of the equity and law of God : the one pretending the cure

The Saint, The Supreme Buddha, is disinclined to action, and to any proclaiming of the Doctrine ".'
Consequently Brahma Sahampati appeared to the Buddha, and addressed him :
' " Reverend Sir, let The Blessed One teach the Doctrine, let The Happy One teach the Doctrine. There are some beings having but little moral defilement, and through not hearing the Doctrine they perish. Some will be found to understand the Doctrine." '
The Buddha proceeds in the narration of his thoughts :
' Then I, O priests, perceiving the desire of Brahma, and having compassion on living beings, gazed over the world with the eye of a Buddha. And as I gazed over the world with the eye of a Buddha, I saw people of every variety : some having but little moral defilement, and some having great moral defilement ; some of keen faculties, and some of dull faculties ; some of good disposition, and some of bad disposition ; some that were docile, and some that were not docile ; and also some who saw the terrors of the hereafter and of blameworthy actions . . . And when I had seen this, O priests, I addressed Brahma Sahampati in the following stanza :
' " Let those with ears to hear come give me credence,
For lo ! the door stands open to the deathless.
O Brahma, 'twas because I feared annoyance
That I was loath to tell mankind the Doctrine." '
—From *Buddhism in Translations*, translated by Henry Clarke Warren, 1922, pp. 339–441).
However much in this narrative may be due to the pious imagination of disciples, there is no reason to doubt that it embodies the fact of a real uncertainty on the part of the newly enlightened Buddha as to his future actions. There is the further interesting parallel between the Buddha's vision of all varieties of people, and the vision of Fox from Pendle Hill of ' the places He had a great people to be gathered ' (*Journal*, p. 60).

of the body, the other the cure of the soul, and the third the property of the people. But I saw they were all out, out of the wisdom, out of the faith, out of the equity and perfect law of God. And as the Lord opened these things unto me, I felt His power went forth over all, by which all might be reformed, if they would receive and bow unto it. The priests might be reformed and brought into the true faith, which was the gift of God. The lawyers might be reformed and brought into the law of God, which answers that of God which is transgressed in every one, and brings to love one's neighbour as himself. This lets man see that if he wrongs his neighbour he wrongs himself ; and this teaches him to do unto others as he would they should do unto him. The physicians might be reformed and brought into the wisdom of God by which all things were made and created, that they might receive a right knowledge of the creatures and understand their virtues, which the word of wisdom, by which they were made and are upheld, hath given them '.[1]

The nature of the ' Truth ' which Fox felt it his mission to declare was determined, largely, by the nature of his experience ; it was this which gave it its distinguishing features. His openings, and later his visions and voices were, in his estimation, derived directly from God, and in no sense mediated through forms, traditions or any other human agency. As it was ' Christ Jesus ' directly commended to him by the uttered voice of God as the only one who could ' speak to his condition ', so it was for all ; and Fox's task became precisely to exhort the people to leave their old dependence upon external forms, traditions, etc., and to direct them

' to the spirit and grace of God in themselves, and to the light of Jesus in their own hearts, that they might come to know Christ, their free teacher, to bring them salvation, and to open the Scriptures to them '.[2]

There are numerous statements of this character :

' . . . I declared Truth amongst them, and directed them to the light of Christ in them ; testifying unto them that God was come to teach His people Himself, whether they would hear or forbear.[3]

[1] Op. cit., p. 17–18.   [2] Op. cit., p. 51.   [3] Op. cit., p. 56.

' I directed them to the divine light of Christ and His Spirit in their hearts, which would discover to them all the evil thoughts, words, and actions they had thought, spoken, and acted ; by which light they might see their sin, and also their Saviour, Christ Jesus, to save them from their sins.[1]

' At another place (in New England) I heard some of the magistrates say among themselves that if they had money enough they would hire me to be their minister. This was where they did not well understand us and our principles ; and when I heard of it, I said, " It is time for me to be gone ; for if their eye is so much to me, or any of us, they will not come to their own Teacher ". For this thing (of hiring ministers) had spoiled many by hindering them from improving their own talents ; whereas our labour is to bring all men to their own Teacher in themselves '.[2]

Summarizing this account of Fox's experience, we find that he grew up in an environment which was full of challenge, and that he faced it with a sensitiveness which caused him to discriminate, at first unconsciously, elements in the situation for definite response to which he was unprepared. At a certain stage of his development these discriminations began to make themselves felt, and consciousness was invaded by depression and anxiety, and the feelings of misery. Other people with whom Fox came in contact, and from whom he sought guidance, were not troubled with any discriminations beyond those special aspects of the times, which could be met along the lines of existing tendencies or systems of tendencies organized in sentiments. This frustration experience, which in many ordinary persons is terminated by the acceptance of an interpretation, or rationalization, provided for them from the tradition of the elders or the authority of spiritual pastors and masters, persisted in Fox for some years. Under the influence of specific shocks, partly contributed from the environment, and partly arising from within (nervous and psychological changes

[1] *Op cit.*, p. 68,   [2] *Op. cit.*, p. 290.

accompanying puberty) Fox began to experience uprushes from the unconscious, first in the form of thoughts, or ideas, dissociated from conscious context, and later of voices and visions, approximating at times to hallucinations ; and through these experiences Fox was able to give form and meaning to the hitherto baffling mystery of existence. But even after this the supreme Reality remained for him something which was ' supernatural ', or ' spiritual ' as opposed to matter for ' notional ' demonstration, and in that sense still beyond the range of the control of the normal tendencies. Truth was, indeed, brought within the range of human capacity to respond to it, since it was inwardly uttered—but it remained essentially mysterious, an operation, gift, or grace of God dwelling in man somehow apart from his natural capacities[1], to be gained, or apprehended by entering into ' the Spirit that gave forth the Scriptures ' and not by any instinctive or intellectual activity. Fox's imaginative interpretation and re-construction, in other words, like all religious interpretation and re-construction, brought the ' beyond ' into relation with human capacities on the condition of an exercise of faith. It still left it surrounded by baffling mystery which could not be resolved, and consequently a matter for religious faith, and not for scientific knowledge. The beyond element was brought into relation with man— but not into a relation which carried with it man's power to control and manipulate ; rather it was the surrender and submission of man in faith to the manipulative control of the mysterious element which characterized the response. That is to say, there still remained an un-

---

[1] Until this inner power came into operation man was ' in the fall of old Adam, in darkness and death, strangers to the covenant of promise, and without God in the world ' (*Journal*, p. 68).

resolvable element in the situation which no terms of cognitive understanding can express, and which can only in any sense be mediated through feeling. Hence the ecstatic language of Fox—in common with all mystics— in trying to describe the indescribable in his experience

' I was ravished with the sense of the love of God. . . .[1]

' Now was I come up in spirit through the flaming sword, into the paradise of God.'[2]

' I saw into that which was without end, and things which cannot be uttered, and of the greatness and infiniteness of the love of God, which cannot be exprest by words '.[3]

[1] *Journal*, p. 27.   [2] *Op. cit.*, p. 17.   [3] *Op. cit.*, p. 12.

M

I have been criticized for the assertion on p. 139 that the 'sensitiveness' associated with creative leadership is a characteristic which 'is at present not reducible to terms of simpler analysis, and must be accepted as fundamental', particularly by Mr. F. C. Bartlett. He, indeed, suggests that my thesis requires a further chapter devoted to the analysis of the 'religious temperament'. Much as I value his judgment and respect his criticism, I am unable in this instance to agree. The expression 'religious temperament' may be taken to imply either (i) a specific drive or tendency, which is the contention of the adherents of the 'religious instinct' theory, or (ii) a plasticity of mental make-up which characterizes in greater or less degree those persons who are not of what Trotter calls the 'resistive' type—a plasticity varying from 'teachableness of mind' to the extreme of abnormal instability. My whole thesis is an attempt to substitute for (i) what I hold to be a truer interpretation of the facts of the religious response than can be expressed by simply postulating a 'religious instinct', and to establish the fact that, from the psychological point of view, religion results from a growing plasticity of mind which breaks down the fixity of stereotyped response. I do not think that much light has so far been thrown on this problem by discussions of the varying 'strength' and general 'arrangement' of the instincts, or by falling back upon secretions of the endocrine glands. At a certain point mind breaks loose from

quasi-mechanical subservience to relatively fixed biological needs. That is, for the interest pursued in this
book, the supremely important instance of plasticity in mental development, and is the source of religion, philosophy,
art and science.   It is a characteristic developed in varying
degrees in different persons, and almost wholly latent
(if present at all) in the typical ' resistive ', while it is
peculiarly marked, as I have endeavoured to shew, in
religious leaders and initiators.   Any adequate investigation
of this characteristic from a genetic point of view yet
awaits to be undertaken, as Graham Wallas makes clear
in his *Art of Thought*.   It will mark a great advance in
psychology when we are able not only to observe the
products and process of constructive thought, but to trace in
detail its embryology and birth.   But we have not yet
reached that stage.

VI

CONVERSION

THE religious experiences of John Rave and George Fox, dealt with at some length in preceding chapters, are instances of the phenomenon commonly known as ' conversion ', and since the general experience of conversion is, or has been, very wide-spread, and not limited to the life history of religious leaders, it is worth while passing in review some of the outstanding features of the process or experience in order to determine to what extent they confirm, or modify, the hypothesis I have been advocating. For this study the researches of E. D. Starbuck[1] are of great value, and will be freely used.

One result of Starbuck's inquiry is to establish the fact that among modern Protestants of America conversion experiences, if they take place, tend in the majority of cases to do so in the period of adolescence. Using autobiographical material specially written in response to a submitted questionnaire, Starbuck drew his conclusions concerning the age of conversion from an examination of 1,256 cases, nearly all of them connected with Protestant Christian churches of America. His general conclusion may be stated in the two extracts here following :

' . . . *there is a normal period, somewhere between the innocence of childhood and the fixed habits of maturity, while the person is yet impressionable and has already capacity for spiritual insight, when conversions most frequently occur* '.[2]

[1] E. D. Starbuck, *The Psychology of Religion*, 4th ed, 1914.
[2] *Op. cit.*, p. 35–6.

It would appear that there is a normal age for conversion at about the beginning of adolescence.[1]

This conclusion is, of course, precisely what might be expected in view of the known physiological and psychological changes which occur at this period of human development. Whether there is a religious experience or not at or about the time of puberty, there is universally a ' conversion ' involving the whole organism, both on the bodily and on the mental sides.

The characteristic thing from the present point of view is the ripening of instincts and tendencies which, while inherited, have not hitherto functioned, and the psychical reverberations which this ripening involves. The responses of the infant life mostly arise from the discharge of self-regarding impulses, and may be said to cluster around ego-satisfaction well into childhood. Indeed, up to the age of twelve or sixteen it is, as a general rule, the case, as Stanley Hall says, that

' . . . the child lives in the present, is normally selfish, deficient in sympathy, but frank and confidential, obedient to authority, and without affectation save the supreme affectation of childhood, viz., assuming the words, manners, habits, etc. of those older than himself '.[2]

J. B. Pratt is even more explicit on this topic :

' The child comes into the world a little animal, and for several years he remains hardly more than a psychological thing. His impelling motives are still chiefly his unmodified and uncontrolled instincts, which play upon him and dominate his life. In fact, we can hardly say that there is any " he ", any self there to be dominated. And the great task of his youth consists in the formation of a true self, which shall be the master and not the tool of his instincts and impulses '.[3]

[1] *Op. cit.*, p. 46.
[2] *Youth, Its Education, Regimen, and Hygiene*, 1922, p. 359.
[3] *The Religious Consciousness*, 1921, p. 122.

This means that the world, for the pre-adolescent child, is a relatively small, confined and definite entity, limited to his own restricted range of response mechanisms, within which his reactions take place easily, unless thwarted by the prohibitions and repressions imposed by authority. But, on the whole, it is true to say that there is a condition of equilibrium as between the tendencies that are ready to function and the main features of the environment that can be discriminated for response. That is, in other words, the situations of childhood are all such as can be met by responses which are rather released by the perceived environment than fashioned by mental effort. Disharmony is due, in the main, to the unwisdom of parents, teachers or guardians[1], and is the result of the arousal of rival tendencies in the child, not of their complete frustration. The child in these years has not been brought into conscious contact with any element of the ' beyond ' character precisely because his capacity for the conscious discrimination of such elements has not yet ripened ; he is not under the urge of any tendencies to action which compel him to become aware of the ' otherness ' in the environment.

I do not propose here to discuss the questions involved in the psychoanalytic doctrine of infantile sexuality. Whether the Freudian formulation is correct or not does not affect the present argument in any vital part. Indeed, the controversy is at least in part a purely terminological one, for few persons, if any, would be prepared to deny that infants display activities and appear to have interests

---

[1] Also, of course, to the repressive influences of a civilisation which requires on the part of its members, even in early youth, a large measure of ' self-control.'

which, if reproduced in an adult, would have a definitely sexual significance. Their significance for the child, as Freud admits, no less than his opponents assert, is not sexual in the sense of 'concerned with reproduction', or in the sense of 'concerned with the conscious perversion of reproductive function'[1] for the simple but sufficient reason that it cannot be. As Dr. MacCurdy says:

> 'It cannot be too often repeated, however, that 'sexual' is too strong a word to use because the child at this time does not and cannot know what the term means in the way an adult does'.[2]

What Freud claims, and claims with justice, is that the facts which he has chosen to call infantile sexuality underlie not only the later development of adult sexuality, but of personality as a whole. But for the purposes of present discussion the important point is not the developmental connection between infantile sexuality and adult sexuality, but the difference, which may be expressed by saying that conscious sex interest enters into the personality as a new factor in the main concurrently with physiological developments which serve it[3]; and the awakening, or activating, of sex interest is one of those psychic factors which brings the growing young person into contact with a widened and deepened environment, which at any point may fade

[1] Freud, *Introductory Lectures on Psycho-analysis*, 1922, p. 266: ' Nor am I at all averse from your thinking the relationship between childish sexual activities and the sexual perversions positively striking. It is a matter of course that there should be this relationship; for if a child has a sexual life at all it must be of a perverted order, since apart from a few obscure indications he is lacking in all that transforms sexuality into the reproductive function.' Also pp. 176, 272-3.

[2] *Problems in Dynamic Psychology*, 1923, p. 294.

[3] This does not seem to be invariable. MacCurdy, *op. cit.*, p. 304, says ' Many young people, particularly girls, may have physiological puberty established without any sex consciousness appearing for years. The same situation is sometimes found among men.' Whether the conscious sex interest develops at physiological puberty or not makes no difference to the point—that when it comes it is a new factor relating the person to a larger environment.

away into mysteriousness. The young person begins to enter upon a phase of life in which frustration becomes possible because of the awakening of tendencies which he does not understand. He has gradually to create and assimilate a new interpretation of his environment and his life before these tendencies can operate harmoniously.

The feature which I have continuously stressed as the genetic factor in religion is disproportion between reactive tendencies and the environment as discriminated. The important aspect here is the excess of discrimination over reactive capacity. It is not a matter of the number, strength, or complexity of the tendencies merely, but of the growth or emergence of the capacity to discriminate something which nevertheless does not of itself act as a stimulus to any one, or any acquired combination, of the tendencies. In all probability the process of this discrimination has an earlier origin than the time of adolescence. It is more than probable that children have received what can only be called ' unconscious ' impressions even in infancy which because they bore no relation at all to existing equipment for response remained entirely unconscious, until they emerged into consciousness, or affected consciousness under the stimulation provided, in part, by the awakening of the appropriate tendencies[1]. Such discriminations can only play any effective part if and when they do directly or indirectly affect consciousness, as happens in the case of certain neurotic symptoms, due

[1] Freud, *op. cit.*, pp. 309-10 : ' . . . it is not at all impossible that a small child, credited as he is with no understanding and no memory, may be witness of the sexual act on the part of his parents or other adults in other families besides those of the proletariat ; and there is reason to think that the child can *subsequently* understand the impression received and react to it.' Jung, *Analytical Psychology*, says : ' . . . there is nothing left but to accept a primary susceptibility of the unconscious, far exceeding that of the conscious ' (p. 85).

to infantile experience, but as happens more normally through the irruption of affect. The maturing of the nervous system is simply the physiological side or aspect of a maturing mental activity which tends to overflow the channels along which it has hitherto adequately functioned. The ripening of an instinct from the point of view of its biological efficiency, may be preceded by psychic reverberations and disturbances which destroy the harmony of the earlier psychic integration on the simpler level. The result, so far as consciousness is concerned, is a kind of psychalgia, which is familiar in theological language as the ' sense of sin ' or the ' conviction of sin '. Starbuck says :

> ' . . . *conversion is a process of struggling away from sin, rather than of striving towards righteousness*. Most of it, as far as our picture of conversion at the present point shows, is worked out in the sphere of undefined feeling, and a relatively small part comes as mentally illuminated aspiration. . . . The evidence in the present discussion is in the fact that the feelings, which are the primal elements in consciousness, function so strongly '.[1]

It should here be noted that Pratt maintains that James and Starbuck have been unduly influenced by the type of ' theologically approved ' conversion, and have arranged their psychology around it.

> ' The theologians (Pratt says) by their teachings have induced a largely artificial form of experience ; and the psychologists coming after, have studied the experience thus induced and formulated its laws, thus making science verify theology '.[2]

There is no doubt a danger here, but Pratt is, I think, mistaken in the view that James and Starbuck have not been aware of it. Indeed, Pratt, in reaction, tends to emphasize it quite unduly. Granted that a typical

---

[1] Starbuck, *op. cit.*, p. 64. [2] Pratt, *op. cit.*, pp. 154-5.

'revival' conversion experience is not a typical puberty experience, so far as its details are concerned, it is still true that the revival experience is one form assumed by bodily and mental disturbances and upheavals which are characteristic of adolescence. What Protestant theologians have done is to provide an interpretation of a particular kind for an experience which is characteristic, if not universal—the experience of turmoil, which is the psychological side of adolescence. They are wrong in so far as they seek to standardize the experience, but the psychologist is not wrong in treating the experience, as affected by the expectation thus created, as being still the expression of mental facts which are far more widespread than this particular form.

The sense of sin which, in one form or another, is so usual in connection with Christian types of conversion, is not necessarily, or even most frequently, related to any actually recognized wrong-doing. Indeed, it is a matter of general observation that on the whole the most saintly characters tend to be most ' conscious of sin '. In analysing and sorting his material, Starbuck found reason to distinguish two typical kinds of conversion, which he describes respectively as the ' escape from sin ' type, and the ' spiritual illumination ' type. Of the latter he says that it

> ' seems to be the normal—at any rate, the most frequent—adolescent experience. It involves a struggle after larger life, and is largely positive, although often accompanied by uncertainty and distress. . . . This latter type is attended, to be sure, with much the same feelings just before the crisis as is the escape from sin, but in this case they are mere incidents to the central fact that the new insight is difficult to attain '.[1]

He further goes on to distinguish the conversion exper-

[1] *Op. cit.*, p. 85.

iences into two groups, (i) *sense of sin*, and (ii) *feeling of incompleteness*, and adds :

'if the cases we are studying are representative, *that type of conversion which is accompanied by the feeling of incompleteness is more common than that which is accompanied by the sense of sin* '.[1]

But in fact the two groups are essentially the same, the difference being due to special features in the environment. The feeling of incompleteness—to adopt this phrase—is the affective state induced by the struggle of ' beyond ' discriminations hitherto effectually kept unconscious, to emerge into consciousness, under the stimulus partly provided by newly awakening tendencies. Granted an atmosphere of evangelical orthodoxy, it is probable that this affect will focus around the idea of sin, and the subject will indulge in fantasies, the material for which is supplied in abundance by Christian mythology. These fantasies engage the activity of the newly-arriving nervous energy, and tend to increase the intensity while defining the quality of the affect experienced. If they can be displaced by other images, suggested through teaching, example, etc., which can act as nuclei for stronger emotions, conversion follows. Or, in other words, if a pathway for the mental activity can be opened up which gives it scope for satis-factory fulfilment, the affective quality will be changed, and the lightness and joy of ' salvation ' will be experienced[2]. But precisely the same mechanisms are involved in the state of incompleteness which does not reach the definite-

---

[1] *Op. cit.*, p. 87-8.
[2] Wm. James, *The Varieties of Religious Experience*, p. 212 remarks : ' There are only two ways in which it is possible to get rid of anger, worry, fear, despair, or other undesirable affections. One is, that an opposite affection should overpoweringly break over us, and the other is by getting so exhausted with the struggle that we have to stop—so we drop down, give up, and *don't care* any longer.'

ness of the sense of sin.   An instructive instance is the case
of George Fox, dealt with in the last chapter.   The affect
is quite as pronounced a feature of the experience as in
cases of conviction of sin, but it is less definite, since it is
not centred upon such fantasies as that of being damned
or lost.   But that the less sharply defined affect is profoundly disturbing is indicated both by Fox, and by
numerous instances quoted by Starbuck[1].   Here again, it
is the opening of a channel along which the maturing
activities can find consciously approved outlet that characterizes the ' new birth '.   Starbuck has admirably
described the process common to both forms of experience
in the following passages :

> ' The facts appear as if, at the time of conversion, there had
> been the liberation of fresh energy, or as if new streams had flowed
> into consciousness.

> ' What shall we say of this awakening of new powers and ac-
> tivities ?   In former years it was said that the person had been
> '' born of the Spirit '', or '' endued with power from on high '',
> a point of view which, from our present standpoint, seems entirely
> accurate.   It is as if brain areas which had lain dormant had
> now suddenly come into activity—as if their stored-up energy
> had been liberated, and now began to function.   The growth of
> consciousness is, in the rough, parallel with the increase of associa-
> tional fibres in the cerebrum, which condition the bringing together
> of the different ideational centres in the brain.   At conversion
> the conditions are as they would be if the various areas were
> suddenly struck into harmony.   If we take into account what
> was observed in a previous section, that those things which now

[1] *Op. cit.*, p. 87 (F. = Female respondent, M. = Male respondent, and the
figures are the age).   F., 15, ' I prayed day after day, struggling for light.'
F., 10, ' The chief trouble was that I did not feel myself so great a sinner
as I thought I ought.'   F., 16, ' I felt the need of a religion.   I read a
certain book and thought over it.   I was beginning to despair.'   M., 23
(this, it will be noted, is George Fox, whose *Journal* Starbuck has included
among his personal responses), ' I prayed and cried to God for help.   I
wandered four years, seeking rest.   I went to many a priest for comfort.
F., 18, ' I felt a dissatisfaction with my way, which lasted several years.
It wasn't guilt.   I didn't know what I wanted.   I had such a desire to be
delivered from sin.'

come into clear consciousness are often the hitherto unnoticed factors in the habitual life, the interpretation seems to be that now suddenly the reflexes in the lower nerve centres are connected by a higher arc with the cerebral reflexes, and so have become elements in clear consciousness. Through the processes of growth, the various brain areas have been lifted to such a potential that they need only to have their equilibrium destroyed to flow into unison, and so bring a flood of latent energy through the new organising centre of consciousness, apparently entirely incompatible with anything that had been present before. *In conversion, accordingly, the new factors may be simply new to consciousness, but factors which had been already latent in the mental life*'.[1]

In terms already employed in earlier chapters of this inquiry, what this seems to mean is that owing to, or concomitant with, the development of the whole organism at puberty, the person experiences the frustration of hitherto adequate modes of response, producing more or less pronounced affect. As the disturbance approaches a climax, active fantasy is induced, which intensifies and specifies the affect, until that image, or imaginal construction, is produced or induced which displaces the painful affect by enlisting the activities of the tendencies in its service, and providing them with satisfying outlets. This means an expansion of consciousness, following the frustration experience, which is a religious experience in proportion as it relates the person to features in the environment which are definitely beyond the manipulative control of intelligent direction. In proportion as the expanded consciousness brings the situation not merely into relation with, but under the practical control or within the verifiable experimental knowledge of, the person, the experience is one of scientific enlightenment or discovery. How the process of the change may be conceived, in physiological terms, is suggested by

[1] *Op. cit.*, pp. 130-1, 132.

Starbuck in a passage dealing with changes analogous to those of religious conversion :

> ' If our analysis of the conditions underlying the change is true, this aspect might be expressed thus : a stimulus, which arouses attention at the same time that it awakens native tendencies of nervous discharge, gives rise to a discharge from the lower reflex arcs into a higher cerebral arc (i.e. awakens an idea). Tension is produced in a new (cerebral) area of the nervous system, which becomes the centre of discharge. Other brain areas, in so far as they are connected by associational paths with this one, likewise bring their contribution to consciousness, so that the whole of consciousness is organised about the new centre, and the entire personality is involved '.[1]

If my contention is true, it should follow that the more a child is kept sheltered in early years, and the less knowledge is imparted to him concerning the unfolding of human life and capacity, and the nature of the real world, the more likely is he at puberty to undergo a ' conversion ' experience of a dramatic kind, since it depends upon the frustration of newly awakening tendencies. The most obvious mode by which a totally ' beyond ' situation may arise and completely baffle the person, is for there to be a maturing of instincts and tendencies which are wholly unexpected and concerning which there is no understanding of their significance. The mind, under these conditions, organized within the relatively simple universe of childish experience becomes like a ship without a rudder, at the mercy of wind and waves ; anxiety, distress, fear, and even terror, may easily be the manner which the irrupting element of ' beyond ' discrimination enters consciousness. And all the imagery of an angry God, a seducing devil, an unforgivable sin, everlasting fire, and so forth, arises to account for, and at the same time to intensify, the psychalgia.

---

[1] *Op cit.*, p. 140.

This, of course, is more especially the case with children who have not only been kept entirely ' innocent ' but have been brought up in a dogmatic and ruthless theological tradition. Many of the older doctrines in their crude form, such as the ' fall of man ', ' original sin ' and ' everlasting punishment ', fit the experience only too well, because they are the product of fantasies born originally out of this experience.

Under the régime of modern educational—and to some extent also religious—ideas and practices the whole tendency with regard to the ' innocence ' of children is changing. The dominant idea now is to save the child from any too sudden irruption into consciousness of utterly baffling elements. Medical men and educationalists have long been urging that sex knowledge should be imparted naturally and gradually to children before they reach the ' storm and stress ' period. Education, in paying attention to the matter of the practical interests of children has largely tended to make possible the gradual unfolding of their capacities and interests in relation to real situations, and in harmony with their own physiological and psychological development. An admirable illustration of the kind of thing is afforded by Edmund Gosse's narration of the way in which his father taught him geography.

' My Father (he says) . . . had a scheme for rationalising geography, which I think was admirable. I was to climb upon a chair, while, standing at my side, with a pencil and a piece of paper he was to draw a chart of the markings on the carpet. Then, when I understood the system, another chart on a smaller scale of the furniture in the room, then of the floor of the house, then of the back-garden, then of a section of the street. The result of this was that geography came to me of itself, as a perfectly natural miniature arrangement of objects, and to this day has always been the science which gives me least difficulty '.[1]

[1] *Father and Son*, Pop. edn., p. 20.

The instinct of curiosity and the tendencies to explore and manipulate were by this means directed into a channel which opened out an expanding opportunity for expression. The principle is that of affecting an easy and imperceptible transition from the spontaneous functioning of the tendencies to their systematic activity in relation to a wider world. Further, as I have already pointed out, religion itself, as an established institution, aims at bridging the gulf between the critical periods, and sheltering the growing person from any too sudden contacts with the altogether mysterious. It has its socially approved and traditionally authorized scheme of imaginative interpretations for most of the experiences of ' beyondness ' which are likely to occur, and it provides the machinery for imparting these ideas and interpretations, as, e.g. the Sunday Schools, Confirmation Classes, boys' and girls' clubs, which all aim, in one way or another, at preparing children for what the Winnebago called life's ' narrow passages '. The Sunday Schools aim at imparting such religious ideas as shall form the nucleus around which the developing tendencies of adolescence can function naturally and easily ; Confirmation Classes, and Church Membership Study Circles aim even more definitely at providing a specific channel through which the inevitable expansion of consciousness can function without involving the turmoil and ferment of any deep ' conviction of sin ' or sense of guilt ; while clubs aim at organizing boys and girls into social groups in which their maturing social tendencies shall find disciplined and harmonious expression. What is done in religious circles by Sunday School teaching, etc., is done outside the confines of established religion in other ways, by the spread of popular information and the inculcation of a popular working philosophy. The result is that the passage from childhood to adolescence is now much more frequently made without any specific crisis—at any rate without any drastic frustration experience. The larger world is entered into and possessed by easy stages ; so much so that it is quite possible nowadays for sophisticated children to pass into adolescence without any recognition of the real and pervasive mysteriousness of life and the universe. To some extent this is furthered by industrial developments which, as Bertrand Russell has observed in his *Prospects of Industrial Civilization*,[1] tends to remove the majority of wage earners from the immediate contacts with the uncertainties of the environment, such, for example, as weather. As a general rule, however, what happens is the gradual discernment of the many aspects of reality which are ' beyond ', and a gradual construction in relation to this discernment of a religious faith which is more reflective, and less purely emotional.

There are two points to make clear. The first is that conversion, in a very broad sense—a rebirth which is both biological and psychological—is a normal, indeed an inevitable experience, and it is characterized by the impingement upon the developing person of a larger and fuller world than that to which he has hitherto been adapted.[2] The second is that the fact that the ' rebirth '

---

[1] 1923, pp. 45-8. ' People who depend upon the weather are always apt to be religious, because the weather is capricious and non-human, and is therefore regarded as of divine origin.' ' The industrial worker is not dependent upon the weather or the seasons, except in a very minor degree. The causes which make his prosperity or misfortune seem to him, in the main, to be purely human and easily ascertainable.'

[2] Cf. William James, *Varieties of Religious Experience*, p. 199 : ' Starbuck's conclusion as to these ordinary youthful conversions would seem to be the only sound one : Conversion is in its essence a normal adolescent phenomenon, incidental to the passage from the child's small universe to the wider intellectual and spiritual life of maturity.'

should take the form of a Christian conversion, with the sense of sin and the attainment of salvation is something which depends not on what is universal, but on quite particular conditions, amongst which by far the most important is the influence of suggestion from tradition, authority and general group expectation.[1] But that this period of life is universally known to be one of critical importance is witnessed to by the widespread prevalence of initiation ceremonies and puberty customs which both mark the gulf which separates the child from the adult, and provide a definite mode by which the transition can be made. Sir James G. Frazer has described a great number of these ceremonies of initiation, which he considers from the point of view of the rites of death and resurrection which are frequently prominent. But as Rivers has clearly stated, rebirth is not always so necessarily connected with ideas of resurrection, and there are many instances of rebirth ceremonies which definitely function as an introduction into adolescence. It may be well to quote Rivers' own words :

'It is necessary in the first place to make clear how I propose to use the term " rebirth ". In anthropological literature the word is used in two different senses. It is used for the process by which a person is believed during life to undergo the process of being born a second time, this kind of rebirth being the central point of a symbolic ceremony. It is also used for the belief that the soul of a dead person is reincarnated in the body of another human being, and in the form which the belief takes most frequently, in the body of one of the descendants of the dead person. I suggest that students of human culture should only use the term " rebirth " when they are referring to the belief in, and

[1] To quote James again, *op. cit.*, p. 200 : ' If they went through their growth-crisis in other faiths and other countries, although the essence of the change would be the same (since it is one in the main so inevitable), its accidents would be different.'

ceremonial representation of, the process of being born again during life '.[1]

It would almost seem as if Sir James Frazer has hardly distinguished precisely enough between these two aspects of rebirth, as the following quotation may indicate :

> ' Amongst many savage tribes, especially such as are known to practise totemism, it is customary for lads at puberty to undergo certain initiatory rites, of which one of the commonest is a pretence of killing the lad and bringing him to life again. Such rites become intelligible if we suppose that their substance consists in extracting the youth's soul in order to transfer it to his totem. For the extraction of his soul would naturally be supposed to kill the youth or at least to throw him into a death-like trance, which the savage hardly distinguishes from death. His recovery would then be attributed either to the gradual recovery of his system from the violent shock which it had received, or, more probably, to the infusion into him of fresh life drawn from the totem. Thus the essence of these initiatory rites, so far as they consist in a simulation of death and resurrection, would be an exchange of life or souls between the man and his totem '.[2]

But what lies behind these ceremonies is something far more fundamental than any supposed pre-occupation with ideas about souls and their possible exchanges. It is the universal experience of the inner and outer changes of puberty. That the symbolism of death and resurrection should play a part, and a large part, is not surprising in view of the fact that the child actually undergoes transformations which lead him to abandon much that has held his interest and to enter into a new and enlarged world of hitherto undreamed of interests. That the child ' dies ' in order that the ' man ' or ' woman ' may be born is a way of expressing the facts which it does not require any mystical initiation to understand. Moreover, the ' resurrection ' is often

---

[1] From Presidential Address, reprinted from *Folk-Lore*, March, 1922, *The Symbolism of Rebirth*, p. 21.
[2] *The Golden Bough*, vol. XI., pp. 225-6.

symbolized as a ' new birth ', as in the case of the Duk-duk association in New Britain :

> ' The boys (Frazer writes) are admitted to it very young, but are not fully initiated till their fourteenth year, when they receive from the Tubuvan or Tubuan a terrible blow with a cane, which is supposed to kill them. The Tubuan and the Duk-duk are two disguised men who represent cassowaries. . . . The Tubuan is regarded as a female, the Duk-duk as a male. The former is supposed to breed and give birth to the novices, who are accordingly looked upon as a newly born '.[1]

This is still more marked in the case of the Akikuyu of British East Africa, who

> ' " have a curious custom which requires that every boy just before circumcision must be born again. The mother stands up with the boy crouching at her feet ; she pretends to go through all the labour pains, and the boy on being reborn cries like a babe and is washed. He lives on milk for some days afterwards " '.[2]

The symbol of new birth, rebirth, regeneration, is indeed so widespread as to have become almost a synonym for the socially approved passage through the puberty period, and the symbol has occupied a quite central place in Christian theology.

The essence of the matter is well expressed by Starbuck in the following words :

> ' Through heredity, doubtless, the brain is endowed with certain structural elements and latent energies which antedate their functional activity. The " sense of sin " is the indication that they are trying to function—that the brute is pressing on to become a man. In its biological significance the sense of imperfection is the price we have to pay for the massive, and at first unwieldy, enlargement at the top end of the spinal cord, which, when mastered and brought into requisition, becomes such a tremendous tool and organ of spiritual insight. The person is restless to be born into a larger world. Finally, through wholesome suggestions, normal development, helped on perhaps by some emotional stress

---

[1] *Op cit.*, pp. 246-7.
[2] *Op. cit.*, p. 262, quoted by Frazer from a letter to himself by Mr. A. C. Hollis.

or shock, harmony is struck, life becomes a unity, and the person is born into a larger world of spirit '.[1]

The fact—whatever its ultimate interpretation may be—is beyond question, that impressions are made on the mind before that which the impressions ' mean ' is so related to interest and capacity as to be able to enter into consciousness, and yet these unconscious impressions, as Freud has said, can be subsequently understood and reacted to. The disturbances which accompany and characterize the changes of adolescence, and which under definite conditions find expression in religious conversion, are of this order. That is to say, they are intimately associated with discriminations which are in excess of equipment, and provide probably the most numerous particular instances of the operation of the fundamental mechanism of the first-hand religious response.

[1] *Op. cit.*, pp. 152-3.

VII

PSYCHOPATHOLOGY AND RELIGION

IN discussing the relation of analytical psychology to poetic art, C. G. Jung laid down the following important principle :

> ' . . . *only that portion of art which consists in the process of artistic form can be an object of psychology, but that which constitutes the essential nature of art must always lie outside its province. This other portion, namely, the problem what is art in itself, can never be the object of a psychological, but only of an aesthetico-artistic method of approach.*
>
> ' A similar distinction must also be made in the realm of religion ; there also a psychological consideration is permissible only in respect of the emotional and symbolical phenomena of a religion, wherein the essential nature of religion is in no way involved, as indeed it cannot be. For were this possible, not religion alone, but art also could be treated as a mere subdivision of psychology. In saying this I do not mean to affirm that such an encroachment has not actually taken place '.[1]

In another place Jung writes :

> ' To our analytical psychology, which from the human stand-point must be regarded as an empirical science, the image of God is the symbolic expression of a certain psychological state, or function. . . .
>
> ' . . . God is not even relative, but a function of the unconscious, namely the manifestation of a split-off sum of libido, which has activated the God-*imago* '.[2]

In the light of this it becomes a pertinent question whether Jung himself has not been guilty of the encroachment he describes and condemns. A further examination of typical references to the religious problem in his writings tends to confirm the suspicion that Jung not only claims the right

---

[1] Paper, *On the Relation of Analytic Psychology to Poetic Art*, British Journal of Medical Psychology, vol. III., Part III., p. 213.

[2] *Psychological Types*, 1923, pp. 300, 301.

to examine the beliefs and symbols of religion as subjective fabrications, which is perfectly legitimate and
necessary, but passes on to philosophical and theological
conclusions of a negative character, which could only be
established, or refuted, by epistemological and theological
discussion. Already in an earlier volume Jung advances
the thesis that the essence of religion is bound up with the
sexual life.

> ' . . . *in essence our life's fate is identical with the fate of our
> sexuality.* If Freud and his school devote themselves first and
> foremost to tracing out the individual's sexuality it is certainly
> not in order to excite piquant sensations, but to gain a deeper
> insight into the driving forces that determine that individual's
> fate. In this we are not saying too much, rather understating the
> case. If we can strip off the veils shrouding the problems of
> individual destiny, we can afterwards widen our view from the
> history of the individual to the history of nations. And first of
> all we can look at the history of religions, at the history of the
> phantasy-systems of whole peoples and epochs. The religion
> of the Old Testament elevated the *paterfamilias* to the Jehovah of
> the Jews whom the people had to obey in fear and dread. The
> Patriarchs are an intermediate stage towards the deity. The
> neurotic fear and dread of the Jewish religion, the imperfect, not
> to say unsuccessful attempt at the sublimation of a still too bar-
> barous people, gave rise to the excessive severity of the Mosaic
> Law, the ceremonial constraint of the neurotic '.[1]

That there was 'fear and dread' in Jewish religion no-
one would deny ; nor the further fact that elements of fear
and dread are present at all times in first-hand religion ;
but on what ground is the fear and dread labelled 'neurotic ' ? The assumption is that the fear and dread were
'false' in the sense that phobias and obsessions are false.
But psychology is not in a position to give judgment on
this issue, on Jung's own showing. It is an encroachment
of psychopathology on the realm of philosophy and theology.
Nor is this an isolated encroachment on the part of Jung's

---

[1] *Collected Papers on Analytical Psychology*, 2nd edn., 1917, p. 172.

psychology. In the *Psychology of the Unconscious* a further step is taken towards the elaboration of a dogma of the pure subjectivity of religion. We are told :

' Just as psychoanalysis in the hands of the physician, a secular method, sets up the real object of transference as the one to take over the conflicts of the oppressed and to solve them, so the Christian religion sets up the Saviour, considered as real. . . . One must not forget that the individual psychologic roots of the Deity, set up as real by the pious, are concealed from him, and that he, although unaware of this, still bears the burden alone and is still alone with his conflict. This delusion would lead infallibly to the speedy breaking up of the system, for Nature cannot indefinitely be deceived, but the powerful institution of Christianity meets this situation. . . . The Deity continues to be efficacious in the Christian religion only upon the foundation of brotherly love '.[1]

This leads on to the assertion that in these days the work of Christianity has really been done :

' The Christian religion seems to have fulfilled its great bio-logical purpose, in so far as we are able to judge. It has led human thought to independence, and has lost its significance, therefore, to a yet undetermined extent '.[2]

The way it has achieved this has been by effecting repressions which safeguard humanity against a dissoluteness in which it could not thrive[3]. We no longer understand the ' feeling of redemption ' which it brought, protected as we are by barriers of its making.

' Most certainly we should still understand it, had our customs even a breath of ancient brutality, for we can hardly realise in this day the whirlwinds of the unchained libido which roared through the ancient Rome of the Cæsars. The civilized man of the present day seems very far removed from that. He has become merely neurotic. So for us the necessities which brought forth Christianity have actually been lost, since we no longer understand their meaning. We do not know against what it had to protect us. For enlightened people, the so-called religiousness has already approached very close to a neurosis. In the past

[1] *Psychology of the Unconscious*, pp. 75, 76.
[2] *Op. cit.*, p. 85.   [3] *Op. cit.*, p. 79.

two thousand years Christianity has done its work and has erected barriers of repression, which protect us from the sight of our own " sinfulness " '.[1]

The implication of this teaching seems quite clearly to be that religion is a device for transference of a peculiarly subjective sort. Ideas are fabricated or accepted which bear no relation to the real elements in the situation, and by virtue of the completely mistaken belief in their validity helpful adaptation is made to the real situation. Since this device relates man to no reality beyond himself and his appetites, when once it has succeeded in its ' biological function ', of setting a limit to the ' unchained libido ', it ceases to have any validity, and its cultivation is by way of being neurotic. Surely this again is an ' encroachment ' on the part of Jung's particular psychology into the domain of what religion essentially is. The discovery of the modes of operation of mental mechanisms involved in the religious response is not the same thing as the discovery of what it is that the response is answering. The psychology of religion has no criterion by which to test the validity of the outer or objective reference of mental processes, and nothing is proved one way or the other by the recognition that mechanisms of ' projection ', for example, are involved in religion. They are no less involved, in one form or another, in most of the characteristic psychological processes. What used to be called ' sensation ' in the static psychology of the past, is now described as ' sensory response '—which involves the recognition of ˃the inner activity initiated by the stimulus, and when we come to the perceptual response, the element of projection is quite definite. Perceptual response means the endowment of a

---

[1] *Op. cit.*, p. 80.

group or system of stimuli with numerous characteristics which they obviously have not got in themselves. It not only interprets the stimuli, and projects the interpretation on the 'external world', but it readily projects upon partial stimulation an overplus of interpretation, a point clearly brought out by Dr. Dawes Hicks in a recent article :

> ' . . . our perception tends to become less and less dependent upon what, at the time, is actually given ; we bring to bear upon what is given a wealth of awareness which ensures that no per-ceptive act is ever, even in its incipient stage, devoid of specific content. Furthermore, it is precisely this wealth of accumulated awareness that constitutes what we are in the habit of describing as our experience ; and in a very real sense it can be said that it is its experience which *makes* a mind '.[1]

But we are not justified on psychological grounds in asserting that therefore the *esse* of a thing is its *percipi*. In the same way, to shew that the mechanisms of projection, transference, etc., are at work in the religious response does not warrant any conclusion, positive or negative, about the existence or nature of the objective reference of religion.

It is to be noted that Jung's illicit conversion of psychology into quasi-theology is largely dominated by the fallacy to which Rivers has drawn attention[2], and which is a particular instance of the fallacy of rationaliza-tion. This fallacy becomes explicit in the passage pur-porting to explain why Christianity was originally accepted :

> ' At this time, when a large part of mankind is beginning to discard Christianity, it is worth while to understand clearly why it was originally accepted. It was accepted in order to escape

---

[1] *On the Nature of Images*, British Journal of Psychology, vol. XV., Part 2, p. 130.

[2] ' One of the fundamental fallacies of the anthropologist . . . is to suppose that because a rite or other institution fulfils a certain utilitarian purpose, it therefore came into being in order to fulfil that purpose.' Quoted above, p. 8.

at last from the brutality of antiquity. As soon as we discard
it, licentiousness returns, as impressively exemplified by life in our
large modern cities '.[1]

Christianity was accepted because in a number of quite
unforeseen and unthought of ways, it actually provided
mankind with a firmer foothold in a growingly mysterious
world. It provided means of release and expression for
activities which would otherwise have been baffled. In
fact, the truer way of stating the case would be to say
that men and women found through Christian ideas and
practices a mode of response which brought harmony into
life, and this was the process of accepting Christianity.
That it also enabled man ' to escape from the brutality of
antiquity ' is not questioned, but that this was the motive
for their acceptance of it is psychologically improbable
to the last degree. Jung is confusing effects achieved
with intentions. No mere recognition of the social dangers
of licentiousness is capable of eliciting of itself a religious
response, nor of persuading mankind to adopt religious
beliefs and behaviour recommended to it as an antidote
to such evils. God could never have been ' invented ',
nor a religious system, such as Christianity, accepted, as
the result of conscious recognition of utility. Something
brings man to the experience of his own inadequacy, and
that something that is ' other ' and ' beyond,' usually gets
formulated in the end as ' God ' (the exception being early
Buddhism). But in all this there is no purposive striving
towards ends of great biological utility. How entirely
this fundamental psychological character of the religious
response escapes Jung, seems to me to be indicated in the
following passage :

[1] *Psychology of the Unconscious*, p. 258.

' I think *belief should be replaced by understanding ;* then we should keep the beauty of the symbol, but still remain free from the depressing results of submission to belief. This would be the psychoanalytic cure for belief and disbelief '.[1]

The essence of religion, psychologically, is the impingement upon human consciousness of that which cannot be understood. What can be understood passes into the heritage of knowledge, and ceases to be impregnated with the emotions that surround the mysterious. Such an extension of the realm of ' understanding ' is constantly proceeding, as I have already maintained ; but its very process involves an ever-deepening awareness of the mysterious immensity, the intellectually baffling ocean of the uncharted ' beyond ' in which all appearances float. As Prof. L. T. Hobhouse has said, reason

' insists as a first principle on the relativity of all human conceptions, on the narrowness of the area reclaimed by knowledge as compared with the ocean of reality, and on the unlimited power of human capacity to expand and explore. . . . We stand on the edge of illimitable, unexplored regions, into which our vision penetrates but a little way. But at least we can dismiss as foolish the fear that science will exhaust the interest of reality, or peace destroy the excitement of life, or the reign of reason cramp imagination. The conquests of mind have a very different effect. The more territory that it brings under its sway, the vaster the unconquered world looms beyond '.[2]

It is always with this vaster unconquered world that looms beyond that religion is concerned, particularly in its manifold relations with that world which has been brought under the sway of reason. Consequently, it is impossible in *religion* to substitute understanding for belief. Religious belief, which can be fully and adequately expressed in terms of scientific understanding, ceases to be religious.

[1] *Op. cit.*, p. 263.
[2] *Morals in Evolution*, 2nd ed., 1908, vol. II., pp. 256-7.

We believe religiously precisely where we cannot understand scientifically. The problem of freeing man from
the depressing results of submission to dogmatic belief
is a very real one, but its solution does not involve the
elimination of belief any more than the solution of the
problem of a headache involves decapitation.

Jung's use of the expression ' the psychoanalytic cure
for belief and disbelief ' leads on to a point of view with
regard to religion which has gained considerable ground :
the point of view, namely, which regards it as essentially
something to be cured.   Reference has already been made
to the idea of religion as a psycho-neurosis[1], but a more
detailed and critical examination of this point of view
will throw light upon the value and the limitations of the
contribution of psychopathology to the psychological
problems of religion, and at the same time may afford
further evidence, or provide further illustration of the
thesis here maintained.   I propose, therefore, to consider
the attempt of Everett Dean Martin, in a recently published volume, to give a systematic interpretation of
religion in terms of psychopathology.[2]

Dismissing the methods of introspection and of behav-
iourism, Mr. Martin proposes to follow a third method
in investigating the ' mystery of religion ', which is

' that of psychopathology. This method is primarily concerned
with the study of abnormal types of behaviour, but it throws
much light upon the psychic life of normal people. There need
be nothing startling in the proposal to study religion as a psychopathic phenomenon. Starbuck and James carried the study into
this field years ago, although their work was done before general
psychology possessed the analytic method of Freud '.[3]

[1] See above, pp. 42-45.   [2] *The Mystery of Religion*, 1924.
[3] *Op. cit.*, p. 47.

It may be well at this point to recall the concluding passages of James's Lecture on Religion and Neurology, lest it should be supposed that his attitude was the same as that of Martin :

> ' As regards the psychopathic origin (James writes) of so many religious phenomena, that would not be in the least surprising or disconcerting, even were such phenomena certified from on high to be the most precious of human experiences. No one organism can possibly yield to its owner the whole body of truth. Few of us are not in some way infirm, or even diseased ; and our very infirmities help us unexpectedly. In the psychopathic temperament we have the emotionality which is the *sine qua non* of moral perception ; we have the intensity and tendency to emphasis which are the essence of practical moral vigor ; and we have the love of metaphysics and mysticism which carry one's interests beyond the surface of the sensible world. What, then, is more natural than that this religious temperament should introduce one to regions of religious truth, to corners of the universe, which your robust Philistine type of nervous system, forever offering its biceps to be felt, thumping its breast, and thanking Heaven that it hasn't a single morbid fibre in its composition, would be sure to hide forever from its self-satisfied possessors ?
> ' If there were such a thing as inspiration from a higher realm, it might well be that the neurotic temperament would furnish the chief condition of the requisite receptivity. And having said thus much, I think that I may let the matter of religion and neuroticism drop '.[1]

What Martin actually intends in his application of the method of psychopathology may be gathered from the following two quite representative quotations :

> ' . . . what if religion were originally fabricated, and its " mysteries " cherished generation after generation, to be an *escape from the very reality* into which modernism would fain confine the objects of religious interest ! ' [2]
> ' *Is it not possible that those unconscious psychic mechanisms which among unadjusted persons find expression in the neuroses, do, under other circumstances appear as religious behavior ?* Religion would appear from this point of view to be a sort of *beneficent psychosis*, or perhaps a socially acceptable substitute '.[3]

---

[1] *The Varieties of Religious Experience*, p. 24-5.
[2] *Op. cit.*, p. 10.   [3] *Op. cit.*, p. 56-7.

The 'real' world is, according to admission, largely extra-rational, and all thinking about it is symbolic—scientific thinking no less than religious and artistic :

> ' As to scientific ideas, their symbolic nature is recognizable when we remember that the " laws " and class concepts of science are really " shorthand " devices, signs by which we are able to indicate that a group of phenomena are similar in a certain respect'.[1]

Nevertheless we are to understand that ' reality ' is too harsh and uncomfortable for man to accept and adapt himself to, and accordingly he distorts it, or ignores it, or accepts substitutes for it, by projecting from the unconscious all kinds of fancies, which roughly represent ' our wish that the universe were run in our interest'.[2] Accordingly, religion is precisely the escape from reality to which reference has already been made. Mr. Martin is very insistent on this point, again and again affirming that the real nature of religion is not that it adapts man to his environment, but that it takes him out of his ' real ' environment, provides him with a means of escape.[3]

But at this point a perplexing problem arises which the author seems entirely to have overlooked. From what ' real ' world is religion a means of escape ? Is it the world of ' everyday experience ' ? But the world of everyday experience is, on his own shewing, steeped, no less than the world of religious experience, in symbolism.[4] Accordingly I must enter a protest against the *petitio principii* involved in speaking of one world of experience as ' real '

---

[1] *Op. cit.*, p. 33. [2] *Op. cit.*, p. 99.

[3] A brief criticism of the ' escape from reality ' theory of religion will be found in my *Psychological Studies of Religious Questions*, pp. 65-8.

[4] Martin gives as instances the use of the map and of the flag as country symbols. ' . . . by the use of the map we are able to *orient ourselves practically* to the reality which we call the United States of America ' (p. 35). ' The flag *orients us emotionally* to America ' (p. 36).

and another as not ' real ' unless some criterion of a specific
kind is offered.   The only attempt to offer such a criterion
is where religion is described as ' nonadaptive ' behaviour.
But to what is it ' nonadaptive ' ?   There can be only one
answer : it is nonadaptive to the realm in relation to
which scientific and practical symbolism is adaptive.   But
it is not necessarily nonadaptive in relation to a realm
which the religious person regards as being no less, but
perhaps rather more real.   The important fact is that the
fantasies projected by religion are not mere escapes from
a ' reality ' which is displeasing : they are constructions
around a reality which is baffling.   Here again the difference between science and religion presents itself.   Both
are constructions around reality.   They differ in the
measure and the nature of the control they give.   Science
is that construction which gives control—using the term
in a broad sense to include the power to foretell.   Only if
the real is equated with the controllable can Mr. Martin's
thesis stand.   The religious man asserts that the uncontrollable, which he is constrained to endeavour to set
forth in image and symbol, is just as real, though it defeats
all his instinctive and habitual modes of response.

In the last chapter of the book, however, the emphasis
is slightly altered ; we are there told that :

' the real trouble is that people *cannot* " *stand themselves* " ' [1]

and that it is not so much the unpleasant or harsh nature
of ' reality ' as the inner turmoil which makes the religious
haven of refuge a necessity.   This, indeed, is the real

---

[1] *Op. cit.*, p. 379.   ' . . . it is not at bottom the world of objects which
people cannot stand.   The real trouble is that people *cannot* " *stand
themselves.*"   It is the struggle for self-appreciation which leads people
to take refuge in a world of ideals.'

text around which the book is written. Man is regarded, religiously at least, as primarily an ' unconscious ' which is the arena of a conflict, because the unconscious is the product of impulses which have been inhibited, thus :

> ' During childhood the individual passes through a long and painful discipline in which he learns to inhibit certain impulses. The environment, he soon learns, necessarily leaves many of his desires unsatisfied. Conscious attention is soon diverted from these impulses and desires. Habits of thinking are cultivated which are in accord with what the environment requires. Thus these unattended tendencies to respond—many of them still being constantly stimulated from within the organism itself— drop out of consciousness. They become the " Unconscious " of psychopathology '.[1]

The mechanisms of religious experience and belief are accordingly exactly those of neurosis, psychosis and dreaming. In fact, it would seem that really it is the ' unconscious ' which ' cannot stand ' the conscious man and his orientation to experience, and it thus takes control, and all unknown to the man himself leads him to harbour images and to cherish ideas and to invent fictions which are simply substitute forms of wish fulfilment. So we find that the Œdipus complex figures as fundamental : a large part of religion is man's attempt to be reconciled with his father image :

> ' As the child approaches adolescence he begins to discover in himself the same force which his childish egoism led him to abolish from the image of the parents. He feels, therefore, that his own maturity is in conflict with the infantile father image through which he now adjusts himself to his world. In the attempt to solve this conflict we see a second and very important function of the father symbol—*the believer must be reconciled to the father* '.[2]

---

[1] *Op. cit.*, pp. 90-1. It is not clear whether Martin means to offer this as the account of the origin of the pathological unconscious, or as the origin of the unconscious which psychopathology has done so much to bring into the forefront of psychological discussion. In either case it is a very fragmentary and incomplete account.

[2] *Op. cit.*, p. 133.

But the mother symbol which appears to be omitted in the formulations of the Deity comes to its own in the religious community. The unconscious desire for the mother can receive symbolic satisfaction in the believer's union with the Church, which is ' mother ' :

> ' The church thus becomes the substitute for the object of that regressive love which would otherwise work serious injury to the psyche. It is consequently a means of grace, it is more than a delightful form of association among like-minded people. Membership in it completes the process of redemption. The symbolism which is used to express this feeling for the church is the language of the " Œdipus Complex " '.[1]

As an instance of the use of this language Mr. Martin actually records the fact that he read or heard that :

> ' a prominent clergyman left one of the large protestant communions a number of years ago, and at the time he left he gave utterance to certain " heretical " opinions in respect to the doctrine and discipline of the church in which he had been brought up. A professor in the leading theological school of the denomination issued a public denunciation of the apostate, saying that he had " slapped his mother in the face " '.[2]

The plausibility of the thoroughgoing psychoanalytic reduction of religion is largely due to the fact that a certain number of religious people suffer from conflicts and repressions which might have led to psycho-neurosis, but have found an outlet and a solution for their troubles in religious forms. The most casual observer of religious phenomena must have noticed how frequently religion has been the refuge of the emotionally thwarted and wounded.[3] Mr. Martin is not wrong in saying that religion

---

[1] *Op. cit.*, p. 241.   [2] *Op. cit.*, p. 239.

[3] In the course of a letter I received recently from a friend—of quite a general character, and not in response to any psychological question from me—she said : ' It seems to me, generally speaking, that the most religious people are the young who are on the verge of manhood and womanhood, and then in mature life, those who have failed adequately to satisfy the emotions in other ways and find what they need in religion and church life.'

is an escape, a consolation, and so forth, *in many instances*, but he is wrong in saying that it came into existence for that purpose, or that this is the essential mark of the religious response. There are psychasthenics in other walks of life beside religion ; but because a woman may find a symbolic satisfaction in nursing in a children's hospital it does not follow that children's hospitals came into existence in order to provide an outlet for the thwarted emotions and instincts of young women who could not otherwise solve their inner conflicts. There is much in Mr. Martin's book which is true and very suggestive Holy Mother Church may often enough be a refuge for the man who suffers from an infantile regression to the Œdipus phase ; but it does not follow that the image of mother was applied to the church because of this unconscious trend in those who founded it. On this ground we might as well say that men who, in later years, speak affectionately of their college or university as Alma Mater really went to college in order to gratify the unconscious incest wish, and that the notion that they went for the sake of education and fellowship was a pure rationalization.

What Mr. Martin succeeds in demonstrating in this book is that once religion had come into existence it probably saved the sanity and mental health of a large number of unstable persons, because they were able to find in it a means of resolving their unconscious conflicts—but, as Freud has shewn, the same may be true of almost any profession. To demonstrate that religion fulfills this, among other functions, is not to account psychologically for religion. The unstable person does not found a religion because he is unstable : he becomes neurotic or even psychotic unless there is something more than an instability which cannot 'stand' the world of everyday reality, or the self of everyday experience. The essential problem of the psychology of religion is those other factors, which provide the positive element in the religious response.

If it were not for his strong pathological bias Mr. Martin would probably have done more justice to facts and considerations which he mentions, but the significance of which he fails fully to appreciate, because they do not fit in with the pathological scheme. It will be instructive to consider some instances of this in which Mr. Martin seems to me to be stating premises, the conclusions of which can only be drawn in terms of the psychological account of religion, which it has been my aim to make some contribution towards outlining. Quite early in the first chapter we are told that :

> ' So large does the mysterious loom in religious experience that it is sometimes regarded as a basic reality in religion. It is said to be that which distinguishes faith from reason. Even so rationalistic a writer as Herbert Spencer seemed to feel that he was giving philosophic validity to the fundamental truth of religion when he maintained the existence of the unknowable, the eternal absolute, and inscrutable cosmic mystery.
>
> ' In very truth the cosmic mystery is ever about us. But I doubt if the mere philosophical fact that we do not and cannot know the ultimate is in itself enough to give rise to a religious appreciation of life '.[1]

But the cosmic mystery is not so easily dismissed as a ' mere philosophical fact '. It may be readily agreed that any philosophical doctrine about the cosmic mystery has little to do with giving rise to a religious appreciation of life ; but the mystery itself, in the concrete ways in which it emerges in various situations, is something very much more solid than a ' philosophical fact '. The mystery is,

---

[1] *Op. cit.*, p. 7.

in truth, an all-environing and unescapable fact, which only grows more and more insistent as man advances intellectually. This is, indeed, recognized elsewhere by Mr. Martin, when he says :

' Perhaps our nearest and truest approaches to reality are æsthetic. Irreducible to formula, the process which we call creation ever eludes the intellect and as pure thinkers we find ourselves in the end always with a mere form of thought. Yet that which we strive to grasp and understand is not an illusion. In it we live and move and have our being. The presence—which we can never escape—we are often aware of as a strange, yet indescribably intimate and immediate, fact of knowledge.

Men have learned to call this mystery of our own and of all existence " God ". The words in which we speak of it matter little ; they are at best but attempts to communicate a fact which is unspeakable '.[1]

The mystery not only communicates itself as a fact in the experience of intellectual defeat, through which the wisest are ever brought to confess that the more we know, the less we understand about ultimate things, but it presses in on the practical and the emotional life no less :

' In one sense (Mr. Martin says), religion is a triumph of faith over pessimism. I believe this pessimism, even defeatism, is always at least unconsciously recognized by profoundly religious persons. Does not Christianity start with the doctrine that this is a lost world, redemption from which is promised through grace?' [2]

It is, indeed, on the practical side that the most impressive lessons of childhood are learned : while so many things can be imagined and thought, so few can be done because of the inexorable, mysterious and baffling limitations that hedge us in. More explicitly yet Mr. Martin seems to me in the last chapter to express precisely those facts of experience which support, not his psychopathic theory of religion, but the theory advanced in these pages. Speaking of the

---

[1] *Op. cit.*, p. 115.　　[2] *Op. cit.*, pp. 64-5.

possibility of a ' revival of religion ', he enumerates a number of conditions which suggest its possibility, and among them this :

> ' There is obviously the fact of our industrialism. It was felt that the invention and use of power-driven machinery would lighten the burden of toil, and in a degree it has done so. But it has also created the modern industrial proletariat, a class of factory hands, gathered in our manufacturing centers not through any natural, mutual attraction on their part, but through the necessities of industry and the demand for labour. These people have been uprooted, torn out of their ancestral environment and are thrown into a mechanically organized world to which they are not adapted. Their old habits do not apply. Their labour processes have been depersonalized and standardized by the machine. . . .
>
> ' . . . All that is quaint, nonutilitarian, picturesque, fanciful, or unique, tends to fall behind and to perish. Human fellowship becomes an unstable equilibrium of forces. And in the degree that men see these forces for what they are, they are going to be unhappy. Labour to-day thinks that it is in revolt against capital. It is really in revolt against the thraldom of industrial processes which under any social system can mean only servitude for the great mass of mankind. As men become aware of this fact—and they must—is it unthinkable that they will seek compensation and escape in religion ? ''[1]

I entirely agree that this describes conditions which are extremely likely to be the prelude to a religious ' revival ', but not primarily, because the conditions described are such as must be ' escaped ' from at the cost of a ' beneficent

---

[1] *Op. cit.*, pp. 350-2. It is interesting and instructive to compare the use made by Bertrand Russell in the passage referred to above, p. 181, of these conditions in his argument about the decay of religion. He considers that the chief reason for the decay of religion is the growth of an industrialism which removes men from close contact with irregularities, such as those of the weather. But his view of religion differs from that of Martin, as well as from that of this book. ' The whole of traditional religion,' he states on p. 47 (*Prospects of Industrial Civilization*) ' may be regarded as an attempt to mitigate the terror inspired by destructive natural forces.' ' The fact is that religion is no longer sufficiently vital to take hold of anything new ; it was formed long ago to suit certain ancient needs, and has subsisted by the force of tradition, but is no longer able to assimilate anything that cannot be viewed traditionally ' (p. 48). Russell—like so many others—is confusing religion with a very special form of religion.

psychosis ', but precisely because they are conditions which defeat existing equipment for response ; and the result of defeat must either be despair and collapse, or renewed effort in a fresh direction.   So far as men find themselves in a ' world to which they are not adapted ', and in which ' their old habits do not apply ', they either adapt themselves intelligently—if the conditions are such as lend themselves to practical understanding and control ; or, in other words, they utilize the plasticity of instinct and habit so as to redirect their activity and thought in such wise as to restore the lost equilibrium between self and environment ; or they must adapt themselves imaginatively if the situation cannot be brought into satisfactory relation with equipment.   Imaginative adaptation may take the form of art, but it is doubtful whether any artistic solution which is not also religious is possible for any but the few individuals who have special aptitudes for artistic expression.   A consciously ' make-believe ' compensation for a thwarting situation can be satisfactory to only the very few : most artists, and all art lovers who find help and joy in art appreciation feel that they are somehow being brought into relation with deeper reality which is ' beyond ' the access of reason, and would echo the words of Robert Browning :

> ' Sorrow is hard to bear, and doubt is slow to clear,
> Each sufferer says his say, his scheme of the weal and woe :
> But God has a few of us whom He whispers in the ear ;
> The rest may reason and welcome : 'tis we musicians know '.[1]

[1] *Abt Vogler*, Stanza xi. Both Mr. Bartlett, after reading the manuscript, and some of my students, after hearing the substance of this chapter in lecture form, raised the question of my view of the difference between art and religion.   I do not feel competent to speak with any authority on the psychology of art, nor is it necessary to my present purpose.   My point here is that religious experience is frequently expressed in the form of art, and that many artists, whether or not they use any conventional religious symbolism, display the essential marks of religion in their work.

From my point of view this is indistinguishable from religion. It involves precisely the same mechanisms, namely, the discrimination of baffling and ' beyond ' elements in the situation and the ' second-thought ' response to them through an imaginative interpretation which still feels them to be beyond intellectual understanding or control. If this imaginative work is wholly fantastic, and a mere ' escape ' from ' reality ', it is not, as I have already argued,[1] religious, but either pathological, or an adult substitute for fairy stories. But if it relates the situation to the equipment of those who have to face it, while inevitably leaving it essentially mysterious, and effectively directs the currents of activity in such ways as to secure the stability and psychological efficiency of the individual and the group, it is religious.

Again in the same chapter Mr. Martin observes :

> ' It is significant that each great mass movement in religion has followed a wave of intellectual advance, and has been the weapon used by the common man in his struggle against a situation which demanded of him too great a readjustment and thus made him feel unconsciously inferior. Christianity follows upon the heels of the Augustan age during which both at Rome and at Alexandria very rapid intellectual advance was being made. . . . The Reformation followed upon the Renaissance, the revival of learning which set Italy in the fifteenth century intellectually on fire and had begun to spread its light all over Europe. . . . English Puritanism also follows the brilliant Elizabethan age, and the " great revival " which appeared simultaneously in England and America at the close of the eighteenth century came as a reaction

I do not contend that all art is religion—a point I endeavoured to make clear on pages 140-142. The artistic response may be (i) a pure ' flight from reality,' offering relief and repose in an admittedly ' make-believe ' world ; (ii) an interpretation of ' reality ' aiming at enhancing its affective value ; (iii) a vision of ' reality ' environed in the unfathomable mystery. It is this third type of artistic response which I regard as being indistinguishable from religion.

[1] See above, pp. 42-5.

against what has been called the most mellow and like unto classic antiquity of all the Christian centuries, the century which spoke of itself as the " age of enlightenment " '.[1]

This relation between intellectual advance and the outburst of religion is precisely what we should expect if the main thesis of this book is correct. Intellectual advance is one part of the process of the fuller discrimination of the larger world, environed in mystery. Every extension of the kingdom of knowledge brings into clearer view the infinite ocean of that baffling mystery. What is to be done about it ? The philosopher may write about it in his intellectual terms, but the ordinary man, under the growing pressure of a universe which again and again defeats him alike practically and intellectually, gathers himself together and by the help of inner resources, fabricates the situation in such images as bring it within the realm of the familiar, trustworthy and friendly—as is illustrated in the case, already examined in some detail, of George Fox. That is the inevitable sequel to any period of advance in intellectual apprehension ; and judging by present day signs I should suggest that the religious revival which Mr. Martin fears is already in process, and that the revivalists are the scientists, who are ever coming upon the mysterious, the baffling, the utterly-beyond, in so various and impressive a fashion that in order to relate themselves to it they are compelled to fabricate it.

And here it will be appropriate to deal briefly with the question of the use of images and symbols. The psychoanalytic ' reduction ' method in religion assumes all the time that any term which is employed metaphorically is not only a symbol, but is a symbol for an unconscious wish,

[1] *Op. cit.*, pp. 370-1.

a repressed and probably discreditable element. Thus if we speak of ' Mother Church ', ' Father God ', etc., we must, according to this teaching, be unconsciously motivated, and any conscious valuation of the terms must be treated as pure rationalization.   And the reason for this is, broadly, that in dealing with the psycho-neuroses analysts have found that the Œdipus complex is often if not always fundamental.   But unless we assume, *ab initio* that religion is a pathological phenomenon, it is at least an equal chance that a metaphor may be a consciously chosen and employed metaphor as that it is primarily conditioned by repressed sexual or other instinctive motives.   Mr. Martin quotes among other Old Testament passages, Hosea ii. 2-4 ; iv. 3-6 ; x. 13-14 ; xiii. 9 ; ii. 19, 20, 23, as illustrating the thesis that

> ' The Hebrews, conceiving of the community in terms of the mother image, " projected " upon the mother the sense of sin which they felt alienated them from the father '.[1]

This is a good instance of the bad habit of assuming that facts confirm a theory without adequately investigating the facts.   We do not know, as a matter of fact, whether the story told by Hosea of his marrying ' a wife of whoredom ' is fact or fiction.   A number of theories about the marriage have been held,[2] and it is just as possible that the prophet actually did marry a prostitute, and seek to reclaim her, as that the story is a parable.   But whether it is experience or allegory, it still remains an unverified assumption that Hosea ' conceiving of the community in terms of the mother image ' is here ' projecting upon the mother the sense of sin ', etc., while the alternative hypothesis that

---

[1] *Op. cit.*, p. 229.
[2] Summarized in A. B. Davidson's Article on Hosea, Hastings' *Dictionary of the Bible*, vol. II., p. 421-2.

the prophet is making conscious use of a personal experience, or of his knowledge of another's experience, in loving and trying to reclaim a fallen woman, in interpreting the moral relationship between Yahweh and his faithless people is, to say the least of it, just as likely. After all, a man's relationship with his wife is largely a conscious one, however much unconscious factors help to determine its character, and as conscious experience it provides manifold points of application to situations which are analogous. For Hosea to depict the community as being like a faithless wife who is yet cared for, and sought with a redeeming love by Yahweh does not involve that he, or in general ' the Hebrews ', were suffering from an unresolved complex which had to issue in the ' beneficent psychosis ' of religion. It means simply that Hosea imaged the Deity as one whose relation to the people had essential points of similarity with that of a devotedly loving husband, whose love was not sexual appetite, but a redeeming passion. And these images are applied to a Deity already formulated, and are in no sense the original projections which constituted the Hebrew conception of Yahweh.

That the sexual instinct and its components play a part, and a large part, in determining the imagery of religion no one would deny : the facts are patent. Once the religious orientation is initiated, it inevitably employs in its work of specific formulation the native and acquired tendencies of man. Thus the nutritive, the herd and the sex instincts all figure prominently in religious belief and practice. Sir James G. Frazer's *Golden Bough* is an extended and detailed commentary upon religion as

' . . . the reverence or worship paid by men to the natural resources from which they draw their nutriment, both vegetable and animal. That they should invest these resources with an atmosphere of wonder and awe, often indeed with a halo of divinity, is no matter for surprise. The circle of human knowledge, illuminated by the pale cold light of reason, is so infinitesimally small, the dark regions of human ignorance which lie beyond that luminous ring are so immeasurably vast, that imagination is fain to step up to the border line and send the warm, richly coloured beams of her fairy lantern streaming out into the darkness ; and so, peering into the gloom, she is apt to mistake the shadowy reflections of her own figure for real beings moving in the abyss '.[1]

But he is careful to add that there is a great deal more in religion than this :

' . . . having said so much in this book of the misty glory which the human imagination sheds round the hard material realities of the food supply, I am unwilling to leave my readers under the impression, natural but erroneous, that man has created most of his gods out of his belly. That is not so, at least that is not my reading of the history of religion. Among the visible, tangible, perceptible elements by which he is surrounded—and it is only of these that I presume to speak—there are others than the merely nutritious which have exerted a powerful influence in touching his imagination and stimulating his energies, and so have contributed to build up the complex fabric of religion '.[2]

In particular Frazer proceeds to refer to the importance of the relations of the sexes to each other, and the influence of ' the forces of attraction by which mankind are bound together in society ' in the development of religion.

But although this is a wider recognition than that of some of the would-be interpreters of religion who see in it nothing but sublimation or distortion of herd instinct, sex instinct or self preservation instinct, it still remains a view which fails to give any account of what is really the main fact. Once religion as a special type of response has been initiated it naturally and inevitably deals with the major interests which man instinctively pursues, but the fundamental problem of religion is : How is it that man comes

---

[1] *The Golden Bough*, vol. VII., Pref., vii.
[2] *Op. cit.*, vol. VII., Pref., vii. and viii.

to pursue these interests no longer directly by instinctive and other controlled practical behaviour, but indirectly by fantasy, imagination, belief, etc. ? A careful scrutiny of the facts of the past, so far as these are available in reliable form, of the facts in connection with the behaviour and beliefs of modern ' primitives ', and of the essence of the processes of our own thought, seems to me to lead to this answer : It is because man is the animal which discriminates more than the isolated presentations for which there is adequate external stimulus, and he does this without having any specific mechanism inherent in his make-up for response. It is this fundamental fact—which itself cannot be explained at present by anything simpler—that lies behind all the mental conflicts, fantasies, daydreams, imaginations, visions, dreams, rationalizations, arts, philosophies, and religions of man. To attempt to derive religion from infantile mental processes is like trying to derive day from night. Infantile processes of fantasy and the rest are themselves the effects of contact with something which is more than the existing mechanisms for response are qualified to deal with. The fate of this ' over-response ' of fantasy depends on various factors and circumstances, which have been in some measure indicated. I may summarize thus : It may be (i) absolutely useless, futile, and non-adaptive. Any person actually trying to behave in relation to such a system would be classified as mentally deranged in any modern civilized community ; (ii) It may be practically effective, leading to symbolical formulations of ' reality ' which enable man more and more to control and to foretell ; (iii) It may be neither (i) nor (ii)—non-adaptive in the sense that it gives no definite control or power to foretell in relation to the mysterious element, but effective in that it liberates the activities, and directs them along channels of behaviour which on the whole do make for adaption to the larger world. The mystery or ' beyond ' is not reduced to nothing, but on the other hand it does not remain the source of mere psychic paralysis, collapse, or aberration. It is so fantasied, imagined and rationalized as to encourage man to continue his process of adaptation to a universe that perpetually baffles, and defeats, and consequently ever calls forth new recognition of the mystery, and further efforts to come to terms with it in imagination and rationalization.

APPENDIX I

RELIGION AND PREHISTORY

In Chapter I the suggestion was made in connection with Mousterian burial practices that it is necessary to guard against the danger of over rationalizing the interpretations of records of prehistoric human behaviour. Nevertheless, it is not too much to say that a new chapter in human psychology has been begun, and some part of it in a preliminary fashion sketched out, in connection with that branch of anthropological study known as Prehistory. From the point of view of the psychology of religion probably the most interesting and suggestive of all palæolithic records of behaviour is that which is preserved in the form of representative and symbolic art ; and it may be at least of interest to raise the question of its possible psychological significance in relation to the theory of the religious response advocated in this book. In the nature of the case any attempt at the interpretation of the paintings, sculpture and engravings of prehistoric man must be purely hypothetical—for reasons already partly indicated. We are dependent for the interpretation of records of behaviour upon arguments of two main sorts : (i) what we think we should have meant under similar conditions by such behaviour, and (ii) what we think modern primitive people mean when, under conditions somewhat similar, they produce similar material. With regard to (i), in so far as we interpret prehistoric art in terms of the ideas and purposes which are dominant in our own conscious relationship with the world, we are liable to the fallacy of rationalization. Nevertheless, if we cannot get back, or down, to feelings in ourselves which underlie our rationalizations, we are not likely to appreciate the real meaning either of the past or the present—a point which is stressed by R. R. Marett :

> ' Where . . . if not close at hand, within range of our personal experience, are we to look for a key to the movement of history ? '

> ' . . . take as another example the fear of witchcraft. Can we not study it among ourselves more effectively than among savages, even though it be written in larger letters on the surface of their lives ? Surely the root-feeling must be apprehended by experience, before its manifestations can be recognized for what they truly are ; and the root-feeling, I maintain, lurks here and now within the breast of every one of us . . . in the penumbra of the civilized mind lurk the old bogeys, ready to leap back into the centre of the picture if the effort to be rational relax for an instant '.[1]

It is therefore only as we are capable of using personal experience sympathetically and emotionally rather than intellectually that we can make any application of arguments drawn from (ii). The person who has experienced quite indescribable emotion on hearing the weird moaning of the wind at night on the lonely moor, and can bring the echoes of such emotional experience with him into the endeavour to appreciate the nature of the savage's responses to things mysterious, is more likely to succeed than the critical investigator who seeks for clear-cut ideas and beliefs behind every religious reaction. But granted the emotional and imaginative power to appreciate the behaviour of modern primitives in these more deep-seated terms

---

[1] *Psychology and Folk-Lore*, 1920, p. 14, pp. 21, 22. Cf. also Sir J. G. Frazer, *Golden Bough*, vol. I., pp. 234-237, where, however, the fact is treated as ' a standing menace to civilisation ' rather than as a help to the psychologist.

of human feeling, the argument from analogy applied to prehistoric man will gain in force and probability.

From the cultural point of view the Stone Age is divided into two eras, Palæolithic and Neolithic. The Neolithic era brings us within measurable distance of historical times, and will not enter into the present discussion. The Palæolithic is again divided into various sub-divisions under the general headings of Lower, Middle and Upper. The Middle period is usually known as Mousterian, from the cave at Le Moustier, where the typical records of this period were first unearthed. The Upper Palæolithic period, with which I am alone concerned here, is divided into four : (1) Aurignacian, (2) Solutrean, (3) Magdalenian, and (4) Azilian.[1] It appears that most of the artistic work of these early times belongs to the periods (1) and (3), the only exception being the ' galets colorés ', which are Azilian. With regard to this artistic work Burkitt says :

> ' Aurignacian and Magdalenian Man, besides manufacturing delicate bone and stone implements, practised an advanced art. This, in all probability, does not apply to Solutrean Man, who apparently had little artistic talent. This art can be divided into two main groups.
> ' 1st. That which is found emblazoning the walls of natural caves.
> ' 2nd. That which is found drawn on bone and stone in the cave deposits, accompanied by dateable stone implements (*Art mobilier*) '.[2]

Some of these paintings and engravings of animals, Burkitt adds,

> ' are occasionally of such beauty and excellence that a modern artist would find them hard to equal. Such an one is the well-known cave at Altamira, where a ceiling in the cave is decorated with paintings, in polychrome, of bison and other animals, before which one stands amazed on thinking of the great gap of time which separates these early folk from us to-day '.[2]

[1] Classification taken from M. C. Burkitt, *Our Forerunners.*
[2] *Prehistory*, 1921, p. 192.

Burkitt enumerates the following among the animals found in cave wall art : bison, ox, horse, and perhaps wild ass, reindeer, stags and hinds, chamois or izard, ibex, elk, mammoth, elephant, rhinoceros, bear, *Felis spelæa*, wolf, fish, birds, and wild boar. He adds :

> ' Human figures always poor, certainly in one case masked ; human hands (negative or positive). . . . Most of the negative hands are left hands, which probably indicates that Man applied the colour with the right hand, being already then a right-handed animal '.[1]

There are also found certain signs, and

> ' These according to their type are described as tectiform, shield-shaped, club-shaped, etc '.[2]

Where these signs seem to be decipherable Burkitt suggests that they may in certain cases represent huts, weapons, traps and conventionalized hands. Regarding *Art mobilier* the same author says :

> ' Man by no means kept his artistic powers exclusively for adorning the depths of caves. Many a fragment of bone, horn or ivory ornament or weapon, from the deposits bears witness to his artistic skill. . . . Though paintings are rare in the *art mobilier*, sculptures, bas-reliefs, and engravings are not so. . . . They are especially numerous in the Pyrenees in Magdalenian times, where an extraordinary number have been found '.[3]

The broad facts, then, are that prehistoric man of the periods of Aurignacian and Magdalenian cultures, carved images and made representations of various objects on implements and tools, and also on cave walls ; some of them of a high order of artistic achievement, others of a more sketchy, imperfect and inferior kind ; and yet others of a highly conventionalized kind, introducing us to the first known examples of symbolism. Among the most frequently represented objects are animals, and the skill of

[1] *Op. cit.*, p. 216.   [2] *Op. cit.*, pp. 216-7.   [3] *Op. cit.*, pp. 222-3.

these primitive artists is declared by competent authorities to be far more evident in their delineation of animals than in their treatment of human figures. Before passing to the problems of interpretation there are certain further facts of interest and significance which may be noted.

(1) There are instances of the representation of the human figure masked. Thus

> ' On the walls of the cave of Hornos de la Peña there is a curious half-human figure. The nose is human, but the leg and arm are hardly so, and there is a tail. In the cave of Altamira once more we have some semi-human creatures, one with hands held upwards as if in supplication, but no legs and a face ending in a snout. Is this a masked human figure ? A seated human figure is engraved in the cave of Combarelles—this time the hand and foot are clearly drawn, and the face and attitude are entirely human. On a *bâton* from the rock shelter Mège there are representations of humans masked as chamois. The feet and legs are human, the body covered with hair and a chamois head and horns in the place of the human head. At the cave of Trois Frères (St. Girons, Ariège) there is the figure of a man (full face) with stag's horns on his head, and a tail. The poise is rather that of the ordinary representation of a kangaroo '.[1]

Burkitt gives a fuller description of this interesting figure in his more recent volume, which, he claims, can only be interpreted in terms of magic :

> ' If the reader will come, in imagination, and explore the cave of Trois Frères, he will see that magic and some sort of ceremonial ritual is the only possible explanation of the wonderful Cave Art. The cave of Trois Frères is in the lower slopes of the Pyrenees, not far from the town of S. Girons. The entrance to it is like a sort of rabbit burrow at the end of another cave called Enlène. For some distance the going is difficult until the passage divides into three. Only a few examples of Art are to be found in the right-hand and middle passages (human hands and punctuations). In the left-hand passage is one of *the most striking exhibitions of Palæolithic Art*. The explorer passes by a small alcove on the right, where under an engraving of a lion a graving tool was found on a projecting knob of rock, probably the actual one used for engraving the lion. Soon after the ground slopes steeply down and ends in a sort of alcove and here we have the most startling

[1] *Op. cit.*, p. 246.

presentment of Palæolithic Art. The vertical walls to the right and left and in front are crowded with engravings of all kinds of animals. There are Bison, Horse, Lion, Mammoth, Reindeer (in all postures), Rhinoceros, Cave Bear, etc. The engravings, which are very well done, occur up to a height which can comfortably be reached by an ordinary man. The wall in front is pierced by a low tunnel on a level with the ground, the hole being quite natural, the result of water action. The engravings continue on the walls and ceiling of this tunnel. Beyond the tunnel the passage turns to the right, and slopes steeply up, to re-emerge as a sort of window overlooking the alcove already described, at some twelve feet above the floor level. Anyone standing at this window dominates the frieze of engravings below, and any crowd of spectators who come to look at these engravings. To the right of a person standing in this window, and at the same level, and so dominating the alcove below, is the figure of a man masked as a stag. The feet are human, but the head has obviously been covered by a stag's mask with antlers. There is also a tail. The figure is partly painted, partly engraved. It can be reached by getting out of the " window " and performing some acrobatic feats. Not only is the figure itself important but its position, alongside the " window " or " pulpit ", dominating the frieze of engravings and any spectators below, is still more important '.[1]

(2) Probably among the earliest objects depicted are human hands, positive and negative. These

' . . . occur at Font-de-Gaume in Dordogne, also at Altamira, in Cantabria, but they are especially frequent at Castillo, near Puente Viesgo . . . North Spain. Here there is a complete frieze of hands. . . . They are also very common (negative) in the cave of Gargas in the Pyrenees, where they have the further peculiarity of appearing to lack some of the end joints of the fingers '.[2]

(3) Among the remains discovered in the Mas d'Azil Cavern and dated stratigraphically as Azilian, were the painted pebbles, or *Galets colorés*, concerning which E. A. Parkyn says :

' These stones are flat and more or less oval in shape, and bear red marks about half an inch wide. Occasionally the whole pebble has been tinted of a rose colour before making the red marks. Often the edge was coloured so as to form a band enclosing the designs, producing a kind of *cadre aux dessins*. . . .

[1] *Our Forerunners*, pp. 208-19.   [2] *Prehistory*, p. 220.

The markings are arranged in a variety of ways, e.g., rows of lines or dots, or they assume shapes suggesting pictographs and symbolical signs '.[1]

Now it is admittedly an impossible task to reconstruct the whole psychology of palæolithic man on the basis of such slender records as these ; but if a complete reconstruction is out of the question it should at least be possible to gain a glimpse into the mental workings of our prehistoric forerunners. The making of designs, whether on objects or with them, or on cave walls, is an act which defies explanation in terms of automatic response to environmental stimuli. Dogs do not make pictures on the sides or tops of their kennels, nor shape out effigies of rabbits, cats, or other dogs. We have here, quite definitely, an indirect and delayed, response, which involves the intervention, between the perception of the situation, and this reply to it, of a mental activity which has imaginatively worked up and supplemented the perceptual features. Is this to be interpreted in terms of a love of art in itself ? Or in terms of a desire for decoration ? Or again in terms of *ennui*, so that the work becomes the result of a mere haphazard passing of the time—as one may, sitting idly on the seashore, make haphazard designs in the sand with the finger or with a stick ? The arguments against any of these interpretations are weighty, at any rate so far as cave wall art is concerned, and may be briefly summarized.[2]

(i) The majority of the engravings and paintings are in the remote depths of caves, where there is no evidence that man made his home. It appears that the entrance of

---

[1] *Prehistoric Art*, 1915, pp. 93-4.
[2] For a fuller discussion reference may be made to Burkitt's *Prehistory*, ch. xxii., and his *Our Forerunners*, ch. x. ; E. A. Parkyn's *Prehistoric Art*, pp. 118 ff. ; R. R. Marett's *The Threshold of Religion*, ch. viii.

caverns and rock shelters were often the home of man, as
is shewn by his ' leavings ', but in such places there is very
rarely evidence of wall decoration.   It is clear that so far
from being decorated dwelling places, the interior recesses
of caverns were resorted to for the purpose of the art
because they were difficult of access and were remote from
the scenes of daily life.   On this point Burkitt says :

> ' We know from the occurrence of deposits containing man's
> implements, traces of fire, bones split longitudinally (man is the
> only animal who does this), that man's home was often in the
> mouth of caves, but there are no traces of his home life in the
> dark, grim, dank interior where he would be boxed in like a rat
> in a trap, by any chance enemy, man or beast, occupying the
> entrance.   It has been suggested that some tectiforms were of the
> nature of constructions where ancestral spirits could live.   This,
> of course, is pure hypothesis, but it is significant that tectiforms
> are often in cracks and fissures difficult of access at the end of caves.
> Niaux is a mile long, with plenty of wall space well removed from
> weathering action, not so far from the entrance, yet no trace of
> art occurs till we reach the extreme end of one of the branches
> some 600 metres from the entrance.   Not contented even then,
> prehistoric man painted one panel of punctuations and signs in
> a sort of alcove in the wall, up to which one has to scramble not
> without a certain difficulty '.[1]

(ii) The nature of the objects depicted—in which animals
bulk so largely—is not the kind we should expect from the
artist for ' art's sake ', but definitely suggests a prevailing
preoccupation with a particular interest.   This becomes
more marked in cases where the animals are depicted as
being wounded, as is the case with bisons at Niaux.   There
are arrows shewn in the side of one bison, and three wound
holes with arrows in the side of another.   Further, the
presence occasionally of masked humans, culminating in
the extraordinary ' man masked as a stag ' of Trois Frères,
clearly indicates that there was a more serious and immediately practical purpose behind the work than that of

[1] *Prehistory*, p. 311.

amusement. Again, there are the tectiforms and other
symbolic signs, whose appearance on the walls, and in the
inaccessible positions mentioned, suggests that they were
regarded as being somehow of vital importance in the life
of man. Speaking of these in the Niaux cave, R. R. Marett
says :

' . . . they could paint up on the walls what they thought,
too. There are likewise whole screeds of symbols waiting, perhaps
waiting for ever, to be interpreted. The dots and lines and pot-
hooks clearly belong to a system of picture-writing. Can we
make out their meaning at all ? Once in a way, perhaps. Note
these marks looking like two different kinds of throwing-club ;
at any rate there are Australian weapons not unlike them. To
the left of them are a lot of dots in what look like patterns, amongst
which we get twice over the scheme of one dot in the centre of a
circle of others. Then, farther still to the left, comes the painted
figure of a bison ; or, to be more accurate, the front half is painted,
the back being a piece of protruding rock that gives the effect of
low relief. The bison is rearing back on its haunches, and there
is a patch of red paint, like an open wound, just over the region
of its heart. Let us try to read the riddle. It may well embody
a charm that ran somewhat thus : " With these weapons, and by
these encircling tactics, may we slay a fat bison, O ye powers of
the dark ! " Depend upon it, the men who went half a mile into
the bowels of a mountain to paint things up on the walls did not
do so merely for fun '.[1]

Finally we have the delineation of human hands, apparently mutilated in the case of the Gargas cave. If the
actual hands were short of the finger joints it is, of course,
possible, as Sr. Alcade del Rio suggested to Dr. Marett, that
' the owners of the imperfect hands were sufferers from
leprosy ',[2] but in view of the fact that Australians and
Bushmen are known to mutilate their hands for religious
purposes, it seems more probable that the same was true of
prehistoric man. In any case, why this representation of
hands at all ?

[1] *Anthropology*, p. 49.   [2] *Threshold of Religion*, p. 216.

' When the explorer examines the frieze of hands at Castillo, and even more the mutilated hands at Gargas, he will have difficulty in explaining them under the headings of *joie de vivre*, or of decoration, and when he comes to sit on the throne of Pasiega, which is partly natural, but partly artificial, on which an implement . . . was found, and looks on the surrounding decorations, if he has any emotion in him he will feel the presence of the sorcerer, who must have sat there in the dim ages past '.[1]

(iii) The man of this artistic age was a hunter, struggling for existence under conditions which, though less rigorous than those of Mousterian times, were still strenuous enough to absorb his ingenuity and activity in the immediate practical tasks imposed by necessity. The time of such mitigation of environmental pressure as would make possible the practice of art not held to be directly useful had not yet come.

Thus it is probable that the real motive for the cave art, and probably for a great part of the *art mobilier* was what we speak of as ' magic ' ; but the implications of the modern conception of magic must not be read back into the primitive mind. The magic response was one which would have seemed perfectly natural under the circumstances as they presented themselves in primitive experience. The question, of course, is : How did the circumstances present themselves ? And the most probable answer to that question seems to be : In such wise as to give the impression that an essential part of them was beyond normal control ; an impression which involves peculiar emotion and generally leads to fantasy, imagination and thought, as we know in personal experience. If we are to bridge the gulf between the time when these primitive hunters sought for food simply under the urge of the food instinct and such acquired tendencies as could be wrought

[1] M. C. Burkitt, *Prehistory*, p. 311.

in under the discipline of perceptual data, and the time
when they added the magical response of trying to increase
their provisions by making pictures and effigies, it can only
be done by the supposition that at some point there was a
felt disparity between the situation presented and the
ordinary modes of adjustment to environment. Nor is it
difficult to recognize the outline of the sort of situation
whose fuller discrimination was the condition for organizing
the magic response. An increasing human horde, and an
ever increasing difficulty in getting enough to eat for the
horde, is a very definite situation, and one which it is not
mere imagination to suppose that prehistoric hunters had
to face. But precisely that situation might face a horde
of animals as a fact, without there being any discrimination
on their part of its crucial features ; that discrimination is,
indeed, a great achievement in mental adaptation, and
carries with it the promise of an ultimate mastery of the
situation. The less adaptable animal, faced with the same
objective situation, but failing to grasp more of it than
presented itself to immediate perception, must continue to
make responses unaffected by the danger or threat of that
which was not only beyond direct control, but beyond its
discrimination. Such animals eat when they are hungry
and can get food, and go hungry and starve if they cannot.
But to discriminate the danger is to be subjected to a challenge, the acceptance of which is the root of all foresight.
The response, in the first instance, to the challenge, was of
a magical order, because no other was possible until
through ages of experimental living, deeper insight into,
and control over reality, was attained.

This does not in any way explain, or aim at explaining,
the origin of pictorial representation. But it does offer a

possible—and, as I think, probable—explanation of its cultivation as an art. The first human being to make a recognizable drawing or outline of an animal may well have done it without any conscious purpose whatever, and his achievement may have been alarming in the extreme to the horde. As Marett says in a similar context :

' Society possibly brained the inventor ; such is the way of the crowd ; but as it duly pocketed the invention, we have perhaps no special cause to complain '.[1]

In the midst, perhaps, of a general uncanny feeling induced by the recognition that the likeness of a bison had been mysteriously made on the ground, or on a piece of rock, there may have been some bold spirit who made practical use of the uncanny presence of bison in the form of its likeness. To control the coming and going of the likeness might be to control the ways of the real bison ; and at any rate a great deal of emotion could be discharged in the ritual of controlling and making and wounding the likeness. Have we not all felt the reverberations of this primitive emotion and its discharge when we have destroyed a portrait or other souvenir of some person in a moment of overwrought feeling ? Thus artistic ability was not originated by a magical idea, but the spontaneous variation in behaviour which was the first dawn of art was assimilated into the culture of the group because it offered itself as a vehicle for the emotion and fantasy already being called into activity by the pressure of an environment in which elements of the strange and ' beyond ' were coming to be discriminated. Once initiated this response maintained itself because of its psychological value. It did not become an alternative to the more direct response to the food

[1] *Psychology and Folk-lore*, p. 241.

situation such as actual hunting, the manufacture of suitable weapons, etc., but it did become an addition, and one which was helpful, not only in giving outlet to otherwise disturbing emotions, but in inducing confidence of success in the business of the chase. A hunter fortified by the expectation of success duly prepared for by the activities of a trusted magician or sorcerer would be far more likely actually to be successful than one who was haunted by the fear lest he should fail to bring back food for the increasing horde of his companions and dependants.

APPENDIX II

A NOTE ON RUDOLF OTTO'S
THE IDEA OF THE HOLY

REFERENCE has already been made to Rudolf Otto's *The Idea of the Holy* (on page 24 above), but the book in certain respects bears so directly upon the thesis I have developed that it requires a somewhat fuller and more critical notice.

In many respects I can appeal to this book for confirmation of the essential features of my thesis. Its chief plea is that while it is a mark of ' high rank and superior value ' in a religion ' that it should have no lack of *conceptions* about God ',[1] or in other words, that it should be rational, yet religion is essentially concerned with a reality or object which ' eludes the conceptual way of understanding ' though it ' must be in some way or other within our grasp.' Religion, in fact, is psychologically based in non-rational processes. It is accordingly a mistake—commonly made— to attempt to ' reconstruct the " bases " or " sources " of religion ' ' in terms of concepts and ideas.'[2] But the account which Prof. Otto proceeds to give of the ' quite distinctive category of the holy or sacred '[3] seems to me to lack psychological completeness, if not validity. He assumes an irreducible religious apprehension, or instinct, while in fact the religious process of a non-rational recognition and construction is capable of further psychological analysis in terms of the frustration of tendencies.

[1] *The Idea of the Holy*, p. 1.　　[2] *Op. cit.*, p. 4.　　[3] *Op. cit.*, p. 4.

If the religious response is absolutely *sui generis*[1] it must be taken as an irreducible datum which may be described, but not analysed. That is tantamount to the assertion, already noted in connection with W. R. Inge (page 15 above) that religion is the expression of an innate and universal disposition, tendency, or instinct. In that case the psychology of religion can only give an account of the various ways in which this fundamental instinct expresses itself in behaviour and belief, and of the manner in which it co-operates with and conflicts with other original tendencies. I have already endeavoured to shew (i) that the religious response admits of a further analysis, and consequently the postulating of an instinct in any specific form[2] is an unjustifiable simplification, and (ii) that the facts of the extreme diversity of the objects to which the idea of the holy or sacred is attached, and the variety of the situations which elicit the religious response, reduce the theory of specific predisposition to absurdity. Accordingly it is one of the first tasks of the psychology of religion to carry its analysis as far back, or down, as possible and not to take refuge in the assumption of an irreducible category. We must be content to lay the foundations before we can rear the superstructure, and much of the present-day psychology of religion is largely vitiated by the neglect of adequate analysis.[3]

---

[1] As seems to be indicated on p. 7, where Otto speaks of a ' numinous ' state of mind which is perfectly *sui generis* and irreducible to any other.

[2] The following quotations shew that Otto makes this assumption : ' a mental predisposition, unique in kind ' (p. 15) ; ' a numinous state of mind ' which is "irreducible' (p. 7) ; ' an inborn capacity ' (p. 63) ; ' an original and underivable capacity of the mind implanted in the " pure reason " independently of all perception ' (p. 116) ; ' the faculty . . . of genuinely cognizing and recognizing the holy ' (p. 148).

[3] I find this exemplified in Dr. W. B. Selbie's *The Psychology of Religion*, 1924.

Prof. Otto analyses the term *holy* into two parts : (i) its moral significance, and (ii) ' a clear overplus of meaning.'[1] It is this overplus of meaning that introduces us to what he proposes to call the ' numen ' ; and the category of value applied to it and the state of mind involved he names ' numinous.'[2] In this terminology, any situation involving the discrimination of features which I have described as having a ' beyond character ' would be one which presented a ' numen ', and the experience of frustration, with its affect and fantasy, would be the ' numinous ' state of mind. Otto's description of the numinous is extremely suggestive and valuable. The question, however, arises whether he has not himself fallen a victim to the tendency he condemns in others, i.e. reading into an elementary psychological reaction ideas and conscious attitudes which are late products of development. Thus ' creature-feeling ',[3] ' the element of awefulness ',[4] ' the element of over-poweringness ',[5] ' the element of " energy " or urgency ',[6] ' the element of fascination ',[7] refer to modes of experience which are *discoverable by rational analysis of the developed consciousness.* To assume that they are ' implicit ' in some elementary numinous state of mind is to attribute far greater clearness and specificity to the first responses to the ' beyond ' or the numinous than fidelity to the known facts warrants. The starting point for religion is in all probability a state of mind quite indescribable in intellectual terms, but most nearly suggested as a sort of aching helplessness. Indeed, Otto

---

[1] *Op. cit.*, p. 5.   [3] *Op. cit.*, p. 8.   [6] *Op. cit.*, p. 23.
[2] *Op. cit.*, p. 7.   [4] *Op. cit.*, p. 13.   [7] *Op. cit.*, p. 31.
                         [5] *Op. cit.*, p. 20.

recognizes this at times clearly enough, as, for instance, when he says :

'Taken in the religious sense, that which is "mysterious" is —to give it perhaps the most striking expression—the "wholly other" (θάτερον, *anyad*, *alienum*), that which is quite beyond the sphere of the usual, the intelligible, and the familiar, which therefore falls quite outside the limits of the "canny", and is contrasted with it, filling the mind with blank wonder and astonishment '.[1]

His further remarks in this regard are important and illuminating. He points out that :

'This is already to be observed on the lowest and earliest level of the religion of primitive man, where the numinous consciousness is but an inchoate stirring of the feelings. What is really characteristic of this stage is *not*—as the theory of Animism would have us believe—that men are here concerned with curious entities, called "souls" or "spirits", which happen to be invisible. Representations of spirits and similar conceptions are rather one and all early modes of "rationalizing" a precedent experience, to which they are subsidiary. They are attempts in some way or other, it matters little how, to guess the riddle it propounds, and their effect is at the same time always to weaken and deaden the experience itself. They are the source from which springs, not religion, but the rationalization of religion, which often ends by constructing such a massive structure of theory and such a plausible fabric of interpretation, that the "mystery" is frankly excluded. Both imaginative "Myth", when developed into a system, and intellectualist Scholasticism, when worked out to its completion, are methods by which the fundamental fact of religious experience is, as it were, simply rolled out so thin and flat as to be finally eliminated altogether.

'Even on the lowest level of religious development the essential characteristic is therefore to be sought elsewhere than in the appearance of "spirit" representations. It lies rather, we repeat, in a peculiar "moment" of consciousness, to wit, the *stupor* before something "wholly other", whether such an other be named "spirit", or "dæmon", or "deva", or be left without any name. Nor does it make any difference in this respect whether, to interpret and preserve their apprehension of this "other", men coin original imagery of their own or adapt imaginations drawn from the world of legend, the fabrications of fancy apart from and prior to any stirrings of dæmonic dread '.[2]

[1] *Op. cit.*, p. 26.   [2] *Op. cit.*, pp. 26-7.

The astonishing thing is that Prof. Otto does not proceed from this to do justice to the psychological implications of what he has expounded in so masterly a fashion. But the trouble is that he is more concerned to establish the ‘objective’ existence of the ‘numen’ and the uniqueness in kind and difference ‘in a definite way from any “natural” faculty’ of the ‘mental predisposition’ which responds to it, than he is to give a psychological account of the ‘numinous’ response. It is not a particular ‘unnamed Something’[1] which stimulates a numinous faculty into activity, as Otto seems to suppose, but it is *anything* which is strange, or ‘beyond’ in the sense of being out of the range of existing tendencies which, being discriminated in its ‘otherness’, brings about the experience of frustration. When this experience of frustration cannot be dissipated by successful control, it suffuses the fantasies and images which are projected upon the inexplicable situation with affect which is an enduring characteristic of the inner side of religious behaviour. All that it is necessary to assume of an original character is the capacity to experience affect, to project images and fantasies, and to discriminate more than can be immediately responded to in instinctive or habitual action. Prof. Otto is dominated by the conception that ‘ *religion is itself present at its commencement* ’[2]—that on no account must it be derived from anything simpler than itself. But, so far as there is any meaning in the expression, it implies that it is fruitless to attempt to analyse the religious response, and that whatever may be the truth of evolution in other realms, it is not applicable to the religious. The result of this

[1] *Op. cit.*, p. 6.   [2] *Op. cit.*, p. 136.

seems to me to be to stifle psychological inquiry and investigation with a philosophical theory. The psychologist who herds and drives the facts in order to round them up into a particular philosophical fold, may get the reputation of being a good pastor, but he is not a faithful scientist. The psychological question here is : Can any account be given of the development of the religious response ? Can we discover and state the psychological mechanisms involved in religious behaviour ? Otto's reply amounts to this : There is a *numen* which lies beyond our rational faculties, but we have a special faculty implanted in us for appreciating and responding to it—the numinous feeling or state of mind. As a starting point for a philosophy of religion this might serve ; the lines of inquiry, based on this as a hypothesis, would then be to determine as nearly as possible what the numen is intended to represent, and to validate the non-rational process by which we apprehend it. Incidentally the problem would have to be faced as to how it is that no common *numen* is universally recognized, but that numinous value is attached in the most varying and conflicting fashion to all sorts of objects, situations and experiences. But to propose this as a psychological explanation of the religious response is like proposing to explain the earth's movement round the sun by saying that the sun attracts the earth to move round it.

The fact is that when man is presented with a situation in which he discriminates the 'wholly other', he is *not* specifically adjusted for response ; and it is this lack of adjustment that originates the religious attitude, and accounts for the extraordinary variety of forms and expressions that it actually takes. The numinous experience is essentially the frustration experience, and not an ' instinctive ' response to a definite numinous object. It is a withdrawal reaction, because there is no definitely envisaged situation to respond to, but a vaguely baffling situation which arouses the peculiar affect which underlies all first-hand religious experience, and is the background of all religious fantasy, imagination and thought.

APPENDIX III

A NOTE ON RESPONSES TO A QUESTIONNAIRE

EARLY in the course of my research I issued a questionnaire on religion[1] which I distributed mainly among university teachers and students, but also to a few other persons. Out of about one hundred copies distributed I received responses, more or less complete, from thirty-five. On so slender a basis I recognize that no statistical generalizations of any importance can be hazarded, and indeed I am doubtful about the value of such generalizations, even on the basis of a large number of responses. The only reason for offering any notes on the answers I have received is that they come almost entirely from persons trained to think, whose considered contributions on the particular questions at issue are at least worth recording and notice.

For the present purpose I propose to make three double groupings of the responses, under the marks A, B and C, as follows :

A Grouping around the first three questions, with special reference to Question 1.

B Grouping around the first three questions, with special reference to Question 3.

C Grouping around Question 6.

The questions with which the A grouping are concerned are :

1. How do you define religion ?
2. Do you believe in God ?

---

[1] The full questionnaire is produced on p. 241 below.

3. Whether your answer to the last question is Yes or No, will you state what you mean by God ?

A Grouping.

I found that the thirty-five responses divided fairly naturally into the following two groups :

GROUP I : Defining religion in terms of God conceived as personal.

GROUP II : Defining religion more generally, and on the whole impersonally.

Fifteen responses fall into Group I, and twenty into Group II.   Typical statements from each group are :

Group I.
    ' The presence of a supreme spiritual power.   Effective contact with some spiritual and superhuman power or powers.   The search for the Other-Self in the Universal.   Belief in the reality of a supernatural power or powers who exercise a controlling and supreme power.   The belief in supernatural beings.   The worship of God.   " The one-ning of the soul with God ".   A dualism in which the non-material is formulated (consciously or unconsciously) as a " Being " or " Beings ".   A personal relationship with God.   Metaphysical beliefs such as the existence of God and of a future life, etc.   Loyalty to, and communion with his creator '.

Group II.
    ' Belief in a purpose in things.   Belief in God who is a sort of transcendental fourth dimension which cannot be understood. A constellation of interests which embraces both my personal ideals and that region of truth which lies beyond my intellectual comprehension.   Depends for its existence on being indefinite. An attitude of one's being towards the life of the world and one's own life as part of it.   Belief in what you think is right.   The attempt to explain himself in terms of the universe, and vice versa.   The ideas of any human being with regard to the purpose of the universe and his relation to it.   A person's attitude towards life.   The organized attempt to express the inter-relationship between ourselves and the Infinite.   An attitude of mind towards the forces which direct the universe and men's destinies.   Attitude of mind which arises from the sincere appreciation of spiritual values.   The reaching out of the human personality towards the unknown and the incomprehensible.   Faith in anything whatsoever.   One's whole attitude to the universe.   Consciousness

of a spiritual value in life beyond the visible and tangible things of every day.   A sentiment in which the mind is directed towards things abstract or spiritual, and away from things material '.

I regard these responses as indicative, not merely of the admitted fact that religion tends to be defined with the utmost variety, but of the further fact that modern religious experience supports the view, here adopted, that however widespread belief in a personal God may be in contemporary religion, it is by no means an invariable characteristic, and that being so it follows that it is a quite arbitrary limitation of the field to define religion in such terms.   Early Buddhism, of course, is the classical example of a religion which had no positive theological formulations ; and I should judge from general observation that the Buddhist attitude to the theological problem is by no means uncommon among modern men and women who are definitely religious.   Dr. Thouless, referring to the question as to

' the particular mark of the conduct, beliefs and feelings . . . which characterizes them as religious ',

considers that

' The man in the street would probably reply that it is the belief in God, and (remembering the existence of polytheistic religions) he might add " or in gods ".   I see no sufficient reason for not adopting this as the distinctive character of religion '.[1]

I suggest, on the contrary, that there is a great deal of evidence that while ' the man in *church* ' would probably reply as Dr. Thouless indicates, ' the man in the street ' will be by no means so reliable, but will, as so many of my respondents have done, define religion without reference to God or gods or supernatural beings sufficiently often to upset Dr. Thouless's own definition.   And from the point of view of the psychology of religion it is surely of first-rate

[1] *Introduction to the Psychology of Religion*, pp. 3-4.

importance to formulate the broadest possible definition, so as to include all types of conduct, belief and feeling which express an identical psychological attitude.

B Grouping.

Three of my respondents definitely do not believe in God in any sort of interpretation. Two of them agree in regarding the word ' God ' as ' quite meaningless '. The third states that

> ' God is the supernatural and supreme power mentioned in (I.) (belief in whom constitutes religion) '.

All three identify religion with belief in God or supernatural powers which they definitely reject. Their responses therefore cannot be expected to yield evidence in regard to the kind of attitude which I have treated as psychologically the essence of the religious response, and accordingly I do not include these responses in the present grouping, nor that under the *C* heading.

The remaining thirty-two I divide into two on the following basis :

GROUP I : Describing God in predominantly rational terms.

GROUP II : Describing God in terms that imply or specifically include reference to a ' beyond ' element which is outside the scope of ordinary apprehension.

Fifteen responses fall into Group I, and seventeen into Group II. Typical statements from each group are :

Group I.
   ' The supreme ruler of the values.'
   ' A person whom I regard as free from a great many human limitations.'
   ' The supernatural and supreme power.'
   ' The supreme power governing and animating the universe.'

' A living being, the creator and sustainer of the universe ; he is timeless and perfectly good. That ever-present, eternal, one and indivisible Being who is Infinite Love, Infinite Wisdom, Infinite Power and Infinite Goodness ; the spirit of truth and source and fountain head of all the divine potentialities in the world and in mankind.'

' A force (internal) leading the individual in the right direction.'

' A power not ourselves that maketh for righteousness.'

' The striving to fulfil that purpose which is inherent in everybody.'

' The one source of power and knowledge and Being—spiritual, everlasting, ultimate.'

' The pervading spirit of love and fellowship which binds human beings together and promotes human welfare.[1]

' The central or focus point of the ideas contained in *my* definition of religion.   (i.e. faith in anything whatsoever [which should lead to what that person would consider " the good "]), i.e. the *purpose* of man's life. Thus by using all our powers and faculties, by attaining self-expression and at the same time making our personalities effective in the world at large we are " attaining to God ".'

' A force permeating the physical universe through which evolution works.'

' A conscious purpose working in all things.'

' The spirit that lies behind the universe and that is linked up with the spirit or soul existent in everyone . . . there is a certain amount of God in all of us, which amount is greater or less according as our spirits are more or less in tune with the infinite spirit. . . . The infinite spirit is, however, a loving spirit, so that there is nothing remote, intangible, cold or unlovable about it.'

Group II.

' The universal spirit, which is more than a person.'

' An eternal Infinite " Being " which caused and maintains the universe, and of which the universe is a part. My ideas are very nebulous, and it is like trying to define the indefinable.'

' Objective deity, non-anthropomorphic, immanent and transcendant, essentially good—in so far as we can understand what is good.'

' God as X, the unknown.'[2]

---

[1] But note that this respondent defines religion as the reaching out of the human personality towards the unknown and the incomprehensible.

[2] The complete answers to the three questions are in this case relevant here :   Religion is a system of beliefs which, shared by a number of people, and evolved (i) to explain man's helplessness against the forces of nature, and (ii) to reconcile the individual to the limitations of his instincts and tendencies imposed by society, have developed a moral code and the worship of a God or gods.   (As to belief in God) :   In God as a spiritual something nterested in the lives of people, no belief ; in God as X, the unknown, no elief or disbelief.

' I don't really know what I mean by God. Some sort of a Power . . . our minds cannot conceive of a God. To try to define God is like attempting to teach a monkey the piano. It is outside his sphere of intelligence.'

' God is the name given to the spiritual power that has the attributes of love, beauty and goodness. These three are the greatest things we can experience, and God is greater than these and beyond our entire conception. He, we believe, understands all that is mysterious to us. God is a sort of transcendental fourth dimension which cannot be understood. He cannot even be said to " exist ", because existence is a logical expression. God only enters into consciousness mystically, i.e. in those rare moments which only the prophet and artist ever experience. These experiences have no relation either to reason or to the emotions and are as indescribable as the Being which is their object. . . . God is a " state of mind ", not a system of beliefs.

' I do not know what I mean by God, though I hope He is someone I can join and form part of.'

' Nature (in the purest sense) plus Love. (This in conjunction with the specific reference in the definition of religion to that region of Truth which lies beyond intellectual apprehension).'

' What is expressed in Browning's
            " God's in His heaven,
            All's well with the world." '

' I find this very difficult to put into words. Matthew Arnold's " Power, not ourselves, which makes for righteousness ", gives a great part of what I should wish to say, but stops short of the whole ; and attempts at definition seem generally unsatisfactory.'

' God simply means to me the explanation (i.e. causes and workings) of natural phenomena which I cannot understand. . . . God simply represents the unknown (i.e. x in mathematics) and if everything were explainable to definite reasons the necessity for x in the equation of the universe would cease to exist.'

' The great ?—the solution of all the riddles of the universe.

' The purpose and constructive force guiding the universe which is beyond our direct knowledge.'

' Absolute Life, Truth and Love indwelling, in reality, in everything, but blurred and misrepresented in the material world.'

' Some great controlling reality behind phenomena '.

The point of interest here is that so many of my respondents should have spontaneously particularized the element of ' beyondness ' in their attitude to religion, and that which they mean by ' God '. It will be noted that the form of the question does not in any way suggest that this was the feature sought for. Regarding the fifteen (or fourteen

—see footnote, p. 235) of the first group, it is impossible to say that they regard religion as definitely a rational construction, for they may well have taken it for granted that the questionnaire was only concerned with beliefs and attitudes of which a rational account could be given, and there may be in all their cases an overplus of extra-rational reference which is unstated.   Perhaps in those cases where religion seems to be identified with ethics (three or four in Group I) it can be asserted that the mysterious element is incompatible with the attitude indicated.   In all the other responses of Group I what is said is consistent with the recognition of mysteriousness, and the emotional reaction to it.   Indeed, it is a question whether all references to the supernatural, the infinite and the eternal, should not have been included in Group II.

C Grouping.

The question with which the C grouping is concerned is :

6. Can you detect any differences between your belief in some scientific generalization which you have not personally verified, and your belief (if you have one) in God, and if so, can you describe the differences ?

The thirty-two responses divide into two main groups on the following basis :

GROUP I : Treating the difference as one of degree of intellectual conviction.

GROUP II : Treating the difference as one of kind, as between rational and non-rational, rational and mystical, etc.

Ten responses fall into Group I and sixteen into Group II.   Of the remaining six three do not answer this question, and three answer too vaguely to be classified. Typical statements from each group are :

Group I.

' A more certain faith in scientific generalizations which I have not personally verified than I have in God, because I can trust that a man makes scientific generalizations on well considered evidence, and there seems no certain evidence of the existence of a God other than a creator.'

' Whereas I am ready to believe second-hand any proved scientific fact—as far as any fact can possibly be proved—my belief in God springs not from what I have been told about God but from some inward conviction. Also I know that my belief in the scientific generalization is open to modification and revision as knowledge of scientific phenomena increases, whereas my belief in God can be subject to no such modification, since God is, was, and ever shall be.'[1]

' The belief in God differs from a scientific generalization because it is essentially personal and is real because we arrive at it through experience.'

' Belief in scientific generalization is belief in authority. Religious belief is belief in something which the particular person has worked out for himself and needs no proof from anyone else.'

' No, except that as it deals more fundamentally with the universe and more nearly with myself than the rules governing the motions of planets, I pay more attention to it.'

' Scientific generalizations are based on proofs other people have made—and I believe those people to be correct. My experience of the progress the world has already made leads me to my religious belief.'

' A belief in a scientific generalization does not usually influence the whole of life. One only acts on it when occasion arises. The only criterion of the presence of a belief in God is a continued attitude of mind, which affects thought and conduct on endless occasions through the day. But if the effect of scientific truths was so personal and important—as in cases where somebody had made it his life's work—there would be no difference. I feel myself that the belief in God involves also a direct dynamic relationship coming from outside oneself, but am not sure that a scientific truth, when it had become personal and important, would not do the same.'

' Scientific generalization has far greater " rigidity " '.

Group II.

' My belief in God is of a totally different order. It is based on immediate spiritual experience. . . . The religious belief em-

---

[1] This response might almost equally have been included in II.

braces the moral and æsthetic sides of my nature as well as the theoretical and is therefore more emotional and active than the other.'

' My attitude to the generalization includes some sort of a realization that I might verify it by ordinary experimental or rational methods. That is absent from my belief in God, so far as I have one.'

' The belief (in God) neither needs nor admits of logical demonstration.'

' I accept (the belief in God) on the basis of my own personal experience, supported by the reported experiences of others. . . . It is not capable of scientific test, neither can it be expressed in an exact formula, nevertheless it is there.'

' Practically, every man, in my opinion, is a mystic . . . and in that case, the two things are totally different. For the former is entirely a matter of intellectual assent ; whereas the latter . . . is also founded upon a mystical (and therefore by definition indescribable) union of soul with God. . . . In believing in God, your assent rests both on your *rational* and on your intuitive experience.'

' Belief in God is mystical and is therefore of an absolutely different nature from scientific belief, which is logical.'

' I know I could verify the one with time. The other is a hope.'

' All the difference in the world. A scientific generalization is at best only a small portion of " Nature ", and is furthermore devoid of love. Likewise belief in God rests (for me) upon experience (personal verification) rather more than upon intellectual conviction.'

' Yes : (a) in the magnitude of the problem, (b) in its unprovability by the same kind of verification as may be applied to a scientific generalization.'

' Belief in God, in a Ruling Power, a Creator, seems to demand more . . . and to be more directly founded upon some need of one's nature which goes deeper than intellectual argument.'

' The belief in God is not, I feel, purely logical and intellectual, it has a strong moral and perhaps emotional element, lacking in the scientific belief.'

' Really to believe in God is not merely to adopt a theory, but to plunge into a life.'

' My belief in God is so largely determined by my own personality and individual relationship to Him that it is my own possession—and has no objective reality, no value apart from myself and for myself. My belief in the sterility of the moon or any other cold fact of science is the intellectual acceptance of a physical fact . . . which exists independent of my acceptance.'

' Belief in God resembles more my belief in a friend than in the so-called laws of nature.'

' I feel the evidence for a belief in God to be different in kind, and in a sense less certain, than that for a well-tested scientific theory. On the other hand I should readily admit that my belief in any scientific theory might be overthrown by new facts, and this would be much more difficult in the case of a belief in God, for the same reason, viz., that no crucial experiment can settle the question one way or the other. I think my belief in God is partly instinctive, and based on the feeling that without it life would lose so much of its meaning and still more of its hope.'

' The essential difference between belief in God and, say, the universal application of the law of gravitation, is that the latter affects only the reason ; the former affects the soul, and is a very large element in the religious sentiment which is dominated and directed by the soul.'

The grouping in this case, as also in the others, is to a large extent arbitrary, for it is impossible to be sure what precisely some of the responses mean. But if I have misplaced any I am inclined to think the balance is overweighted in favour of Group I, and there is unquestionably a preponderance of view that belief in God is primarily a non-rational matter, however much it may become rationalized. That is, the weight of the evidence—for what it is worth—supports the general view of my thesis, that the religious attitude is essentially connected with that which is beyond the sphere of rational control and foresight.

In view of the discussion as to the existence of a religious ' instinct ' (page 15 above) the responses to the question (7d), ' Is religion the expression of a specific instinct ? ' are of interest. Out of thirty-five, twenty reply No ; five reply Yes ; four state that it depends on definitions ; two say they are doubtful ; two reply probably not ; one replies probably (yes) ; and one does not understand the question.

THE QUESTIONNAIRE

For the purpose of an Inquiry in the Psychology of Religion Questionnaire issued by J. C. Flower

WILL you please answer the following questions as briefly as possible ?

1. How do you define Religion ?

2. Do you believe in God ?

3. Whether your answer to the last question is ' Yes ' or ' No,' will you state what you mean by God ?

4. Does the word ' God ' tend to call up any image or images in your mind ? If so, please describe ; if not, can you give any account of what does happen mentally ?

5. What does religious faith mean to you, and what essential marks do you consider necessary to constitute religious faith in another person ? (Faith as an attitude, not as a system of beliefs).

6. Can you detect any differences between your belief in some scientific generalization which you have not personally verified, and your belief (if you have one) in God, and if so, can you describe the differences ?

Please answer the following questions by ' Yes ' or ' No ', with any necessary comments :

7. *a.* Is religion invariably characterized by some reference to the supernatural ?

   b. Must religion involve a felt practical relationship with what is believed in as a superhuman being or beings ?

c. Can there be religion in the absence of belief in and
    reference to God or gods, or the supernatural ?

d. Is religion the expression of a specific instinct ?

e. ' Religion is an organized system of instincts, ten-
    dencies, emotions, and ideas, which exercise a
    dominant influence on belief and practice, and
    determine them in the direction of the discovery,
    preservation and increase of value.'   Is this
    definition :

    I.   Too broad ?
    II. Too narrow ?
    III. Scientifically adequate and precise ?

*   *   *   *   *   *   *

Any personal information respondents are willing to
give will be valuable, especially Age, Sex, Department of
Study, or Predominant Interests, Religious Attachment,
etc.

INDEX

TO AUTHORS QUOTED AND REFERRED TO

GENERAL INDEX

Printed and bound by CPI Group (UK) Ltd, Croydon, CR0 4YY

01/11/2024

01782635-0003